GW00601874

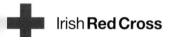

Irish **Red Cross**

CARERS
HANDBOOK

A practical guide to looking after someone
who is ill, elderly or has a disability.

The Irish Red Cross is part of the International Red Cross Movement.
Registered Charity Number CHY 3950

Irish Red Cross second edition reviewed and amended by

Ellen Keane	Chairperson Community Services Working Group
Mary Rose Day	Lecturer in Public Health Nursing
Dr. Andrew Kelly	Chairman Medical Advisory Working Group
Bernie Stevenson	National Training Manager
Lucy Banks	Services Support Officer
Catriona Finn	Youth and Services Assistant
Elaine Monaghan	National Services Support Officer
Gavin Lane	National Services Assistant
Ronan Ryan	Head of Fundraising & Communications

The Irish Red Cross would like to thank the following for their help with producing this book:

The staff and management of the Centre of Education, Beaumont Hospital
The staff and management of Mount Carmel Hospital Dublin
Lydia O'Halloran - IRC Community Services
Marie Harte - Registered Nurse
Catherine Kilmartin - Public Health Nurse
Photographic models, Kathryn O'Halloran, Lydia O'Halloran, Jason Southcombe
and Niamh Southcombe
National Florence Nightingale Committee of Ireland

First edition, entitled Helping you to Care Handbook, published in 2007 by the Irish Red Cross
Second Irish edition published in 2013 by the Irish Red Cross

Adapted from *The Carer's Handbook*, first published in Great Britain in 1997 by Dorling
Kindersley Limited, 80 The Strand, London WC2R 0RL

Publisher's note: the type of information in this publication is subject to regular change.
Readers are therefore strongly advised to seek independent verification that any
particular procedure reflects best practice, at the time they seek to apply it.

ISBN 978-0-906077-16-0

16 Merrion Square, Dublin 2, Ireland

t +353 (0) 1 642 4600
f +353 (0) 1 661 4461
e info@redcross.ie

www.redcross.ie

MESSAGE FROM PRESIDENT HIGGINS

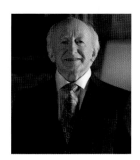

It gives me great pleasure to welcome you to the second edition of the Irish Red Cross 'Carers Handbook'.

This publication follows on from the very successful first edition of the handbook which was a practical and useful resource for almost 10,000 carers. Carers play a vital role in looking after the most vulnerable members of our society. Those who take on the role of carer, often without any formal training, may feel overwhelmed and vulnerable themselves. This handbook provides practical support and advice for those looking after someone who is ill, elderly or has a disability.

The level of attention and care given by family carers could not be matched in our health care system and therefore I fully support any initiative which provides support to them - such as the practical information provided in the handbook. While we all have within us the ability to care, an informed carer will provide a better quality of care and a happy safe environment for both the recipient and the carer.

I wish to congratulate all of those involved in the publication of this second edition of the Irish Red Cross' 'Carers Handbook'. I am confident that it will continue to be a valuable aid to those who require support and guidance in the tireless work they do as carers.

Michael D. Higgins
President of Ireland
Honorary President of the Irish Red Cross

CONTENTS

DISCLAIMER

The information supplied is believed to be correct at date of publication. This should not be relied upon as a substitute for appropriate medical or legal advice. In certain circumstances it may be necessary to contact medical or legal professionals or other appropriate services.

INTRODUCTION

More and more people are being cared for at home, partly because hospitals discharge patients more quickly and also because people live longer. There are a large number of carers in Ireland looking after an ill, disabled or elderly person at home. This is an illustrated and practical guide to address their needs.

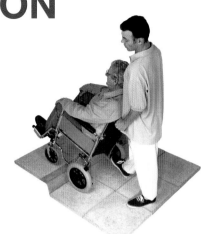

BEING A CARER

People become carers for different reasons. You may have chosen to look after a relative at home because he or she has come to depend on you and you do not want him or her to live in a residential home or hospital. Alternatively, you may be a volunteer carer, who has chosen to give up your own time to provide help in the community. **Carers are crucially important to the person they look after providing a range of assistance.** Whatever your situation, this book will give you the information and guidance you require so that you can provide the best and most rewarding care.

This book outlines - and aims to complement - the support that you can expect from Health and Social Services. We strongly suggest that you make the most of this help and any financial benefits. Access to the right information, support and resources can help you to improve your quality of life and that of the person you are caring for.

THE PERSON YOU ARE CARING FOR

Care needs can vary greatly. Some people may require only a few weeks of help while they recover from an illness or an operation. An elderly, disabled or very ill person, however, may need dedicated care for many months or years. Whoever you are caring for, your aim should be to provide care without depriving the person of his or her independence and dignity.

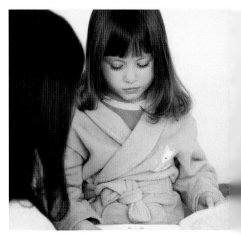

HOW THIS BOOK CAN HELP YOU

This definitive guide to home caring offers practical advice, emotional support and essential information to help you provide the best quality of care possible.

Practical advice Step-by-step photographs show you the best ways to carry out daily activities such as communication, personal hygiene, nutrition and mobility.

Emotional support The emotional difficulties that both you and your relative may face are addressed and solutions are offered to help you overcome some of these difficulties. Reassuring advice is offered to guide you through distressing situations.

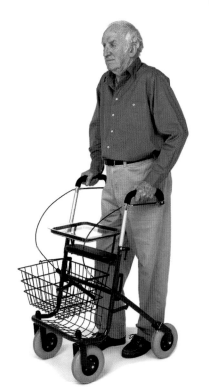

A GUIDE TO THE TERMS USED

Gender: throughout the book, we refer to the person being cared for as 'he' or 'she' alternately from chapter to chapter, except in text that relates directly to an image.

RELATIVE	The person being cared for. We use this term as most people are related to the person they are caring for. The information in this book, however, is equally relevant if you are caring for a friend or a neighbour.
HOME CARER	Any person caring for a relative, friend or neighbour in the home environment.
VOLUNTEER CARER	Any person working as a carer for a voluntary organisation.
CARE/ HEALTHCARE PROFESSIONAL	A member of the professional care team. The chart overleaf gives details of the professionals and the services that they provide.

CARE PROFESSIONALS

The chart below outlines the professionals with whom you may come into contact while you are caring for your relative. The actual job titles may vary from region to region; the possible alternatives are given in brackets. A care professional that is clinically trained, such as a GP, Public Health Nurse or Occupational Therapist, is known as a 'healthcare professional'.

CARE PROFESSIONALS AND WHAT THEY DO

CARE PROFESSIONAL	LOCATION	SERVICES PROVIDED
GENERAL PRACTITIONER (GP)	GP Practice/ Health Centre	A doctor who provides a wide range of general medical services to their patients on an ongoing basis with the option of referral to medical consultant when necessary.
PRACTICE NURSE	GP Practice	Involved in all aspects of patient care for example health promotion, smoking cessation and vaccination programmes.
PUBLIC HEALTH NURSE	Community based / Health Centre	Advice and support to mothers before and after delivery, and also on child health & development. Delivery of school health services. Provision of personal nursing care to the elderly, persons with disabilities, patients who have been discharged from hospital. Advises on equipment. Support services for carers in the home. Provision of appropriate referral service.
SOCIAL WORKER	Community based/Health Centre Community based/Hospital	Assesses the needs of adults and children. Produces a care package and guidance on how to obtain services.
OCCUPATIONAL THERAPIST	Health Centre /Hospital	Assesses a person's individual requirements and advises on adapting the home, equipment and activities to enable him/her to achieve their optimal potential and independence and where possible self-sufficiency.

CARE PROFESSIONALS AND WHAT THEY DO

CARE PROFESSIONAL	LOCATION	SERVICES PROVIDED
PHYSIOTHERAPIST	Hospital/ Community/ Health Centre	Treats those with bone, joint and breathing problems. Advises on mobility and exercise following assessment. Ante/Post natal care.
CHIROPODIST	Health Centre / Hospital / Home Care / GP Surgery	Offers specialist treatment and therapy for foot problems.
SPEECH & LANGUAGE THERAPISTS	Hospital/Health Centre/Community /School	Provides services to children and adults with communication and/or swallowing difficulties.
DIETICIAN/NUTRITIONIST	Hospital/ Health Board	Advises on a healthy diet; tailors special diets to suit specific medical conditions, such as diabetes.
PALLIATIVE CARE TEAM	Hospice/Hospital/ Community	Provides care for those with a terminal condition, including pain and symptom control. Offers advice and support to patient's family and carer, including organising short-term respite.
CONTINENCE ADVISER	Health Centre/Hospital	Provides advice and support for those with continence problems.
DIABETIC LIAISON NURSE	Hospital/ Community	Advises on the effective control of diabetes and overall health.
STOMA CARE NURSE	Health Centre/Hospital	Provides advice and support for a person who has a stoma.
INFECTION CONTROL NURSE	Hospital	Advises on prevention and control of infection.
AMBULANCE PERSONNEL (EMTs, PARAMEDICS, ADVANCED PARAMEDICS)	Ambulance Station	Provide pre hospital emergency care and transport for patients.

Other Support Services include: Care Assistants, Home Help and Meals on Wheels.

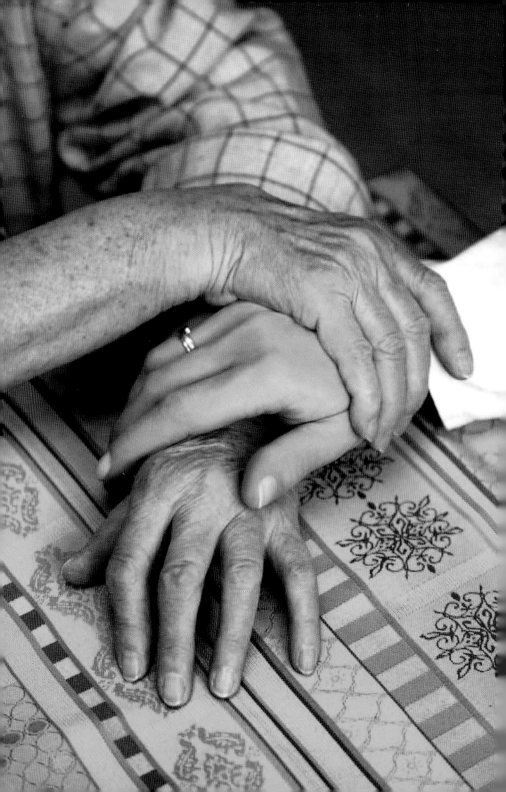

CHAPTER 1

BEING A CARER

The decision to provide care at home for a relative who is ill, elderly or has a disability is not one to be taken lightly. Although caring for someone can be very rewarding, it can also affect your home and family life, your work and your free time. If your relative has gradually come to depend on you, you may have become a carer without realising it. In this situation, it is still important to decide whether it is the best option for you.

This chapter outlines aspects of being a carer, so that you can weigh up the advantages and disadvantages of looking after your relative at home and make an informed decision about becoming a carer or continuing to be one. It may also help you to accept that caring at home may not necessarily be the best option for you and your relative. If you do reach this decision, your GP and Public Health Nurse should be able to advise you on alternative care arrangements.

LOOKING AFTER YOURSELF

To be able to fulfil your role as a carer you need to maintain your own physical and emotional health. To achieve this, you need to ask for help and take time off when you can. This section shows how you can take advantage of the help that may be on offer - from friends, family, Social Services and voluntary organisations. Asking for, and accepting, help can enhance your relationship with the person that you are caring for.

BECOMING A CARER

Your role as a carer, and the length of time it lasts, can vary. If your relative's decline is gradual (as with Alzheimer's disease), caring may be something you are prepared for; but if his decline is sudden (due to a stroke, for example), you may be quite unprepared for looking after him. Whatever the level of care, make sure it is the right choice for both of you.

THE LEVEL OF CARE

Your relative may be self-sufficient in many ways, but unable to cope with tasks such as shopping or cleaning; this could mean that he only needs your help for a few hours each week. In more extreme situations, however, you may be looking after someone who requires help with basic needs such as bathing and feeding; in these circumstances, you would be required to provide constant care.

LONG-TERM CARE

If your relative's physical or mental abilities are permanently impaired, you should seriously consider the practicalities of caring for him at home. In most situations quite extensive care needs will have to be considered. Full-time care may be required and may involve adaptations being made to your home - for example, a stair lift may have to be installed, or a downstairs room may have to be converted into a bedroom.

SHORT-TERM CARE

A person recovering from an operation or a major illness will require a high level of care initially. A care plan outlining your relative's needs should be prepared with advice from the GP and Public Health Nurse. If there is any task you think you cannot cope with, you should tell the hospital, your relative's GP or Public Health Nurse. At first, you may be required to help with day-to-day tasks such as cooking or, if your relative has mobility problems, to help him to get from room to room. As he recovers, however, your responsibilities should decrease. Someone who has had a heart attack and is convalescing at home, for example, may require intensive support and care initially, but will gradually regain his strength.

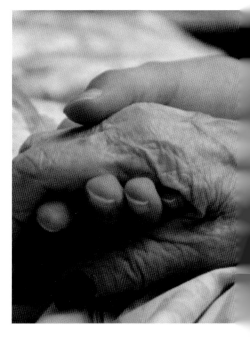

IS HOME CARE A PRACTICAL OPTION?

Caring for a relative can be a big responsibility that may affect nearly every aspect of your life. It is essential to have your care situation assessed by a Public Health Nurse so that you can consider your own needs and those of your family and relative. Remember, home care is not the only option available to you: if you have doubts, there are other practical alternatives. Before deciding whether to become a carer, or continuing to be one, consider the questions below.

YOU AND YOUR RELATIVE

- Will your relative require long or short-term care?
- Will he need constant supervision?
- How does he feel about you being his carer?
- Are you the best person to be his carer?
- How much help can you get from friends, family, voluntary agencies and Social Services?
- What other options are available if you don't become the carer?

YOUR PARTNER & CHILDREN

- How will others in your household be affected?
- Can you fulfil your responsibilities to your relative, as well as to your partner and your children?
- Have you discussed the situation and made the decision as a family?

YOUR HOME

- Will you need to adapt your home?
- If so, will the changes be expensive? Are you eligible for grants?

WORK AND FINANCES

- Is it possible to get short-term compassionate leave, or carers leave?
- Are you prepared to give up your job, if necessary?
- Will either of you receive benefits?

REASSESSING YOUR DECISION

Your relative's condition may improve or decline over time, affecting his level of dependence on you. Symptoms and circumstances change continually; remember, your first decision need not be final - you can reconsider some of the above factors at a later stage.

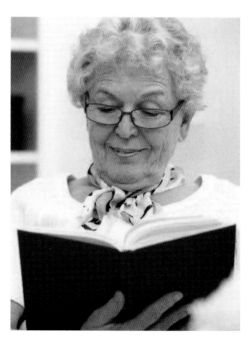

BENEFITS OF HOME CARE

Although being a carer is never easy - and there may be times when you feel greatly challanged - it can be a most rewarding and satisfying experience. There will be demands and challenges to rise to, and you may find that you are forced to draw on previously hidden reserves of strength. Caring can also be a fulfilling experience as you see your relative benefiting from the care provided.

BENEFITS FOR YOU

Your role as a carer is ultimately one of giving, but do not forget that there are also benefits for you.

Emotional strength Your relative is likely to rely on you for comfort and support when he is in low spirits and in need of reassurance. You may find that the emotional support you provide strengthens your relationship, bringing you closer together.

Pride You should be able to take pride and satisfaction in the fact that your relative is receiving the best care that you can provide.

Organisational skills Looking after another person requires you to learn to prioritise and organise your time efficiently; these skills can stand you in good stead throughout your life.

BENEFITS FOR YOUR RELATIVE

You are uniquely placed to provide your relative with a quality of life that may not be possible elsewhere.

Independence You can plan your time and structure a typical day together. This will give your relative a level of control and freedom that he may not get in a more ordered environment, such as a residential home.

Personal care The smallest things, from knowing the type of soap your relative prefers, to preparing his favourite meal, can make an immense difference to his quality of life. Maintaining some semblance of normal home life may be very reassuring for him.

Comfort Being cared for at home means that your relative is in familiar surroundings, close to the people and things he knows and loves. He may be reassured to know that you are close at hand to lend emotional support whenever he needs it. He may also want to be close to a pet, such as a dog or cat.

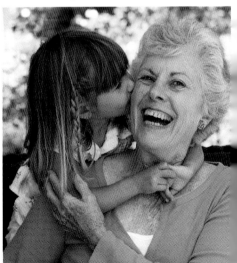

HOW RELATIONSHIPS CHANGE

Caring for someone can affect your relationship with that person and other people to whom you are close. When someone who was previously fit and healthy becomes dependent because of an illness or disability, power balances shift and roles within a relationship inevitably change. By the same token, some relationships are fortified by the intimacy and closeness that caring brings.

CARING FOR YOUR PARENT

Most of us look up to our parents and rely on them for love and support, even when we have families of our own. It can be very distressing for you when the person you have always relied upon becomes frail or ill, and you may feel that you should assume the responsibility for looking after him. When a parent's health deteriorates, we are all reminded of our mortality. In such situations, role reversal is inevitable but not easy for anyone to accept. It may be difficult for a parent to accept that he is no longer the protector and provider, and must look to you for care. You, on the other hand, may feel you are being pressured into a caring role, and feel guilty for wanting to avoid the responsibility. For many, however, caring for a parent becomes an opportunity to repay them for their help over the years.

CARING FOR A CHILD

When a child becomes severely ill or has a disability, he or she may not have the same opportunity as other children and this can cause overwhelming grief. Your instinct will probably be to overprotect your child but, where possible, you should encourage him to learn to do things for himself. Contacting a specialist organisation to learn about his illness or disability, and the limitations it will impose, may help you to cope. For example, with the right support, a child with specific needs may develop skills that will enable him to lead a full life. The specialist organisation may also be able to put you in touch with other parents caring for children who have the same illness or disability.

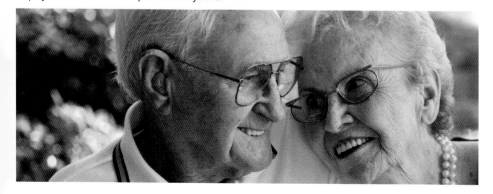

CARING FOR YOUR PARTNER

Most couples entertain a romantic dream of growing old together. Whether sudden or gradual, the transition of one partner into being a carer brings inevitable change within a relationship: one partner needs to provide more care and support while the other becomes increasingly dependent. It may be a difficult time and you may both have to learn to cope with feelings of sadness: you because the person you love is ill; your partner because he has to adjust to this new, unexpected role of being a dependant.

COPING WITH TASKS

When an illness is physically debilitating, you may have to minister to your partner on quite an intimate level. This may bring you closer together, but you may also find it awkward and embarrassing and want to consider enlisting outside help.

UNDERSTANDING YOUR FEELINGS

If your partner has an illness that affects him mentally, such as Alzheimer's disease, for example, there may be times when you feel that you have lost sight of the person you fell in love with, and become frustrated and angry because you can no longer communicate as you used to. There may even be times when you feel hurt, insulted and angry because your partner becomes confused and does not recognise you. These are natural feelings; if you become exasperated, speak to someone who can understand.

ADAPTING TO A CHANGED SEXUAL RELATIONSHIP

It may be that your partner's illness has changed him physically and that this has affected your sexual relationship. If so, it is important that you share your feelings openly. He may feel ashamed or awkward, and, if he senses that you are becoming distant, it will only reinforce his feelings of isolation. Sex is an important part of a relationship, but people are often shy about discussing it, worrying in silence rather than seeking advice. Sexual desire does ebb, and at times your levels of desire may not be compatible. If you and your partner cannot talk openly, ask your GP to recommend someone who can help.

THE EFFECTS ON YOUR FAMILY

If your relative comes to live with you, try to involve your partner and your children in his care. This will ease some of the strain on you and will also help your relative to feel that he is part of the household. Your family may be affected in different ways.

Children They may feel neglected, even jealous, especially if you are having to devote more of your time to your relative and less to them. Try to make time for them and, if they want to, involve them in helping you to care for your relative.

Partner Make time for your partner; he/ she too may feel neglected. Try not to take out your frustrations on him or her, and be as honest and open as possible with each other: hiding your feelings will put an unnecessary strain on your relationship. Your sex life may be affected: the physical and emotional exhaustion of being a carer can in itself be enough to reduce sexual desire. Discuss this with your partner and give reassurance that your feelings have not changed.

LOOKING AFTER YOURSELF

As a carer, you have responsibilities to yourself as well as to the person you are caring for. Looking after your physical health and being conscientious about your own diet, taking time off, exercise and sleep will keep you strong and help you to maintain your emotional resilience. If your health begins to suffer, you will not be able to help your relative or yourself.

DIET

If you are busy and your relative has little appetite, you may be tempted to skip proper meals and exist on snacks. Consider the suggestions below as ways of finding time to enjoy a meal:

- Regularly invite a friend or relative over for a meal. This will provide a break, as well as some company; it may also inspire you to prepare a meal.
- When inviting a friend, or even a group of friends, suggest that everyone contribute a dish to the meal.

EXERCISE

Even though you are physically active as a carer, you should try to make time for regular exercise away from home. This will make you feel more energetic, and provide a break from your daily activities. Try to find the most suitable exercise option.

Exercise classes A class can provide a regular break in your routine; it may also be refreshing to meet people not involved in caring. Can you set aside a block of time each week and be sure that you can keep to it? Could you arrange for a friend to sit with your relative for a couple of hours while you attend a yoga class? Could you go to an exercise class while your relative is at a day centre?

Swimming and walking Time wise, these activities are much more flexible and demand a lower level of commitment than classes. Although more solitary, it may suit you better just to switch off and swim a few lengths of the pool or go for a walk in the park.

Exercising together Is there any way your relative could accompany you to the sports centre? Some local pools run swimming classes for people with disabilities; this may be a way for you to exercise at the same time.

DO'S & DON'TS

Looking after yourself is an essential part of caring for someone else. • **Do** get enough sleep. • **Do** discuss any plans for dieting (with a view to weight loss) with your GP. As a carer, your energy requirements may differ from someone else of your age and build. • **Do** drink plenty of fluids, especially water. • **Do** eat plenty of fresh fruit and vegetables. • **Do** moderate your alcohol and cigarette consumption. • **Don't** use alcohol or cigarettes as a crutch in stressful moments. • **Don't** snack on cakes and biscuits to maintain energy levels. • **Don't** forego proper, regular meals. This is easy to do, but is not good for you in the long term.

UNDERSTANDING EMOTIONS

Caring can be emotionally draining, and you may not always be able to maintain a positive outlook. There may be times when you are confused by your feelings, even ashamed, but the worst thing you can do is to bottle them up. The first step to understanding your feelings is to identify them; it is only then that you can find ways of working them out.

IDENTIFYING STRESS

It is difficult to avoid becoming stressed; you may often feel that there are not enough hours in the day and that there is no end in sight to the jobs you have to tackle. You may become irritable and moody and feel constantly tired. You may find that on some days even the simplest of tasks, such as the washing up, is just too much to handle. By identifying the signs of stress early on and dealing with them, you can limit their destructive effects.

RECOGNISING AND OVERCOMING STRESS

When you recognise the first signs of stress, try the following stress-reducing tips:

- Breathe in deeply and slowly through your nose and out through your mouth. Repeat ten times.
- When you are offered time off, use it to spoil yourself. Try not to think about household tasks you could be doing. Get out of the house: visit a favourite place, see a film, have your hair done or visit friends.
- If you can't get out, have a long, relaxing bath with essential oils or bath salts. Read a magazine or listen to your favourite music.

- Ensure that you go to bed at a reasonable hour, if possible, and that you get enough sleep.
- Try to take some exercise during the day. If you can't get out of the house, is there an exercise programme on television or DVD/video that you can do? Gentle exercise, such as stretching, may be good for both you and your relative, and may be something you can do together; it may even be a source of laughter.
- Talk to someone about how you are feeling and, if it helps, have a good cry. A friend, your GP, a Public Health Nurse, a specialist organisation or support group may be able to listen and help.

ALLEVIATING TIREDNESS

There is nothing more likely than tiredness and exhaustion to fray your temper and make you irritable. Think about ways in which you can alleviate tiredness.

Planning your day Draw up a list of your typical daily tasks, then prioritise them. Are they all absolutely necessary? Could you delegate some of them to family or friends? For example, could someone else do the ironing while you have a short rest?

Getting adequate rest If your relative sleeps in the afternoon, you should try to nap then too. If you have trouble getting to sleep at night, the following tips may help:

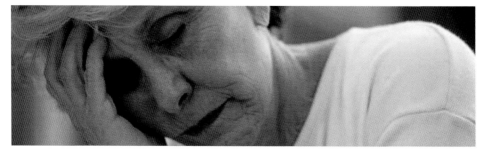

- try to keep to a regular bedtime routine;
- keep the bedroom at a comfortable temperature;
- avoid stimulants such as caffeine before bedtime;
- don't go to bed hungry.

- you feel that the situation is unjust, that neither you nor your relative deserves what is happening;
- it may be an expression of the frustration you feel as a carer; you may simply feel that you cannot cope.

UNDERSTANDING ANGER AND GUILT

It is only human to feel angry when something happens that hurts you or upsets your plans. This is a natural and healthy response, especially when someone you love falls ill or becomes disabled. Anger is a complex emotion, often suppressed because we feel guilty about expressing it. If you can get to the root of your anger, you will have gone part of the way towards dealing with it, and also with the accompanying guilt. There are certainly times when anger needs to be controlled, but it should never be ignored. Here are some of the more common reasons why you, as a carer, may experience anger and guilt:

- someone you love is suffering;
- the illness or disability has upset all your future plans together, and you feel guilty about feeling angry;
- you feel angry with your relative for being ill and, even though you know this is irrational, it does not stop you feeling this way;

DO'S AND DON'TS

Anger can get out of control and lead to irrational judgements and decisions, even violence.

- **Do** discuss your problems with the GP or care professional; either may be able to refer you to someone who can help.
- **Do** seek the help of a specialist organisation that has knowledge of your relative's illness; they will be able to empathise with your situation and offer you and your relative advice and support.
- **Do** get away from your relative for a few minutes if you feel yourself becoming tense. First, make sure he can be safely left on his own.
- **Do** try to understand that your relative may feel angry and frustrated at times. He may also feel guilty about having to rely on you so much.
- **Don't** cut yourself off from friends because you are angry with them for not sharing your suffering. You will only isolate yourself further and become embittered.
- **Don't** be ashamed of your anger. Talk about your feelings before they become overwhelming.

COPING WITH LONELINESS AND ISOLATION

It is easy to become isolated as a carer. You may find that you are too busy to keep up with friends and relatives. If people visit less frequently, it may be because they see that you are busy, and worry that they may be in the way. Sometimes people stop visiting because they are embarrassed about your relative's illness.

The following positive steps may help:

- make time to contact people and reassure them that you still need their friendship and support;
- try to be open and honest about your feelings and your needs - don't shut people out or try to pretend that you can cope on your own. To feel happy in your caring role you also need to feel supported and loved;
- be open about your relative's illness and what it means in terms of daily care;
- offer reassurance to people if they are frightened or upset by the signs of the illness - remember that they are not as familiar as you are with the situation;
- enlist the help of friends and relatives, and involve them in the care if you can. People are often happier if they know they are making a positive contribution.

RECOGNISING DEPRESSION

There may well be times when everything gets on top of you, when you don't know where you will find the resolve to go on. Normally these feelings will pass if you talk to a friend, get a good night's sleep or take a break. Sometimes, however, they persist and develop into depression, which can be destructive. Some of the more common symptoms of depression to watch out for are:

- tearfulness;
- irritability;
- tiredness;
- feelings of inadequacy;
- lack of concentration;
- fitful sleep with early morning waking or too much sleep;
- eating all the time, or complete loss of appetite;
- lack of motivation and interest;
- low / depressed mood.

If you are experiencing any of these symptoms and you feel that you can't discuss your feelings with a friend, you might want to consider seeking impartial advice from a counsellor or GP.

SEEKING COUNSELLING

Carers often face problems that seem insurmountable.

Can counselling help?

Counselling is one way of helping people adjust and come to terms with their difficulties; it is also good for exploring practical ways to solve problems. Counselling is not a 'cure' for people with psychiatric or physical illnesses and it is not psychotherapy, which is a treatment for people with specific mental health problems.

Choosing a counsellor

Your GP should be able to advise on a suitable counsellor.

FINDING TIME FOR YOURSELF

Looking after someone full-time is a demanding job. At times you will need a break, not only from daily chores, but also from your relative, for either a few hours, a day, a week or longer. To do this you will need respite care. Respite care ranges from someone sitting with your relative for an afternoon or your relative going into a residential home for a short stay.

MAKING TIME FOR YOURSELF

You may feel guilty about wanting to have a break, feeling that it implies that you do not care about your relative. However, there are many reasons why it is essential to take time away from caring.

To reduce stress levels Being stressed will mean that you are more prone to illness, irritability and depression. Carers often soldier on unaided, denying themselves any relief until their own health suffers. Time away can help you to put things in perspective.

To improve your caring relationship To keep a relationship alive and interesting, you need to talk to other people and have other experiences. The relationship that you have with your relative is no different: time apart will almost certainly give both of you new perspectives and different things to talk about.

For your independence Your relative is necessarily dependent on you, the carer, but remember that you also need care, not least in the form of emotional support. Spend time keeping up with friends and family and maintaining your own social life. Try to carry on with a hobby, if you have one. Retaining some degree of independence will mean that you are less likely to become isolated and feel overwhelmed.

RESIDENTIAL RESPITE CARE

If you are thinking of taking a break for a week or more, one option is for your relative to go to stay in a community hospital/nursing home. Consider the following when you are choosing a temporary care home:

- Is it registered with the Health Service Executive?
- Are the staff experienced in dealing with your relative's particular needs?
- Does your relative like the place?
- Is it well-kept and clean?
- What is the food like?
- Are the staff friendly?
- Are temporary residents fully integrated into the life of the home?
- Can they participate in activities?
- Are there others having a temporary break?
- Is it comfortably furnished?

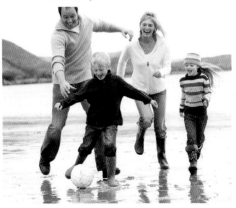

RESPITE CARE

The best type of respite care for your relative will depend on his particular requirements, the length of time you will be away and the cost involved. Cost and availability will vary according to the area in which you live. If you require only a short break, it may be worth asking family and friends for help in caring for your relative.

TYPE OF CARE	LENGTH OF BREAK	SERVICES PROVIDED
DAY CENTRE	A day or more a week, as required.	This will vary from centre to centre. Services such as chiropody and hairdressing may be available as well as a range of social and other services.
HOSPITAL	As required.	Complete medical and nursing care, including rehabilitation.
HOSPICE	According to requirements, it could be from days to weeks.	Pain and symptom relief, spiritual support, counselling service and alternative therapies, such as massage. Home visit service may be available.
NURSING HOME	Convalescence 1-2 weeks.	This will vary from home to home, but may include occupational therapy, chiropody and hairdressing.
RESPITE	1-3 weeks or weekends or a few days at a time.	

HOW CAN FAMILY AND FRIENDS HELP?

Some people will be keen to help but may be unsure as to exactly how. Here are some suggestions:

- Could someone sit with your relative for a few hours to give you a chance to rest or go out?

- Could a member of the family come and stay occasionally, or could your relative go and stay with him or her?
- Could someone help with the ironing, hoovering, laundry or washing up?
- Could anyone help with small tasks such as shopping or picking up a prescription?

LEVEL OF CARE	WHERE TO FIND OUT WHAT IS AVAILABLE
From attendant to registered nurse, but it depends on staffing levels and whether or not people who have certain conditions are catered for.	Health Services, Voluntary organisations, GP's surgery. Contact the Public Health Nurse at your local Health Centre.
Doctors and registered nurses. Specialist help, such as physiotherapy and occupational therapy.	Referral from GP.
Full care with specialist doctors, registered nurses and complementary medicine specialists.	Referral from GP, Public Health Nurse. Admittance normally limited to those with cancer or those who have a terminal illness.
Usually care assistants, registered nurses with additional medical cover by GP's.	Referral from GP, Public Health Nurse, family, support groups, voluntary organisations.

GOING ON HOLIDAY TOGETHER

Caring for your relative does not mean that you have to be permanently confined to the home. Respite holidays enable your relative to have a holiday - in the care of someone else - thereby also affording you a break. If you want to go on holiday together, there are several organisations that arrange holidays for those with special care needs.

CHOOSING A HOLIDAY

Holidays that cater specifically for the needs of people who are ill or have a disability are available: these provide different levels of care depending on individual needs.

Planning ahead

Make sure you discuss any special needs and the level of care required with the tour operator beforehand. Most can offer useful information, such as the location of purpose-built holiday centres and whether or not there are carers on hand to assist with daily care, such as helping someone to eat.

Getting there

A local voluntary aid organisation may be able to assist with travel arrangements, such as transport to and from stations and airports, or the travel company itself may be able to organise this. Most rail companies offer help, and airlines may give assistance and help at airports, to people who have mobility problems.

FACILITIES CHECKLIST

Before booking a holiday, check that the facilities are suitable for your relative's needs:

- Is there wheelchair access to all areas - to the dining room, gardens and lifts, for example?
- Is the accommodation accessible to someone with limited mobility? Is your relative's room on the ground floor, for example?
- Is there a lift/stairlift?
- Are there facilities for people with disabilities, such as handrails in the toilet, bathroom and shower?
- Are there bed and bath hoists?
- Are there bed lifts/different bed heights?
- Are there facilities for guide dogs?
- Are registered nurses, care assistants or trained medical staff available?
- Are treatments, such as physiotherapy or hydrotherapy available?

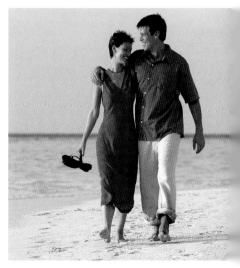

SUPPORT GROUPS

People who share experiences of a particular type of illness or disability often form groups so that they can offer support and understanding to each other, and share tips on how to cope. There are two types of support group: those formed to provide information about a particular condition, offering help to you and your relative, and those that are there to support the carer.

WHY JOIN OR FORM A SUPPORT GROUP?

By joining or forming a support group you can benefit from meeting new people in a similar situation to yourself and offer and receive help and advice.

To meet others in a similar situation

The life of a carer can be a very isolated one: meeting and sharing your experiences with others in the same position can be life-affirming in itself.

To have a break

It is understandable to want time away from your caring role. Support groups will often find someone to sit with your relative, and may be able to arrange transport to and from the meeting.

To obtain information

If an illness is rare, and experience in dealing with the symptoms is limited, support groups can provide an opportunity for carers and their relatives to meet and pool their knowledge. These groups often offer specialist training as well. Support groups can also keep you up-to-date regarding benefits and your rights as a carer.

For support

Members of the groups are usually carers, ex-carers or have direct experience them-selves, so are well placed to understand your problems and offer practical advice and support. Because they are or have been in your position, they will be able to identify with your feelings and reassure you that you are not alone.

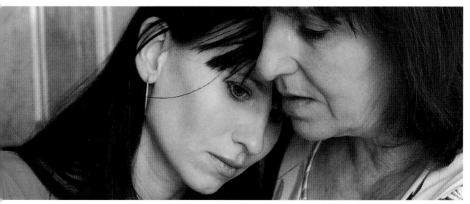

ARE YOU COPING

It is possible that you and your relative may find that home care is not practical. While many adapt easily to the role of home carer, some, understandably, find it difficult to cope. Bear in mind, too, that circumstances may have changed and it may be time to look at alternatives for care. It is important, however, that you are both happy with the final decision.

ASSESSING YOUR SITUATION

To find out if home care is still a practical option for you, examine your day-to-day routine and consider how you are feeling physically and emotionally.

Organisation Is there a routine to your day? Are you managing your time as efficiently as possible?

Priorities Are you wasting time and energy on unnecessary tasks and problems that will only increase your stress levels?

Support Are you getting all the help you can? Have you considered all your options: friends, relatives, voluntary organisations, Health and Social Services?

Financial entitlements Are you claiming the benefits to which you are rightfully entitled?

Physical health Are you eating and sleeping properly? Are you able to exercise on a fairly regular basis?

Emotional health Are you able to maintain a rational outlook? Do you feel on top of things at most times? If not, do you have a friend or a counsellor with whom you can share your feelings?

Breaks Are you getting enough time for yourself? Are you taking regular weekly breaks or holidays?

Independence Can you get out to see friends? Do you still have a social life?

Commitments Can you keep commitments to others in your family and to yourself?

A PERSPECTIVE ON YOUR DECISION

If at any stage you decide that you can no longer care for your relative at home, do not feel guilty or think that you have failed. It will probably be in the best interests for both of you if he is provided with alternative care, especially if he needs more specialised help and supervision than you are able to provide.

CHAPTER 2

BEING A VOLUNTEER CARER

A volunteer may be required to look after a person if there is no friend or relative to act as a carer. A volunteer may also be required to help a home carer; either to allow him or her to take time off or to help him or her with strenuous tasks that he or she cannot carry out alone, such as helping his or her relative to get out of bed or into the bath. Health and Social Services increasingly rely on voluntary organisations and the volunteer carers who work for them, to provide both short and long-term support.

THE ROLE OF THE VOLUNTEER

As a volunteer, you may be supervised and supported by a care professional, such as a Public Health Nurse, who is responsible for assessing the needs of the person and who will advise you on the level of care that is required. Integral to your role is the ability to get on with people - the person being cared for, the home carer, if there is one, and the professionals with whom you may work. In order to provide the best service, you should feel fulfilled in your role, which means being able to address problems and ask for help when necessary. Being a volunteer can be hard work and is sometimes very challenging, but ultimately it can be a highly rewarding and satisfying experience.

BECOMING A VOLUNTEER

People of all ages can volunteer to become carers: voluntary organisations, such as the Irish Red Cross, welcome the help of anyone who is willing to give up time to assist others.

WHAT DOES IT INVOLVE?

Becoming a volunteer carer may be a daunting prospect for many people. Below are some of the most common questions asked by potential volunteers.

WILL I BE INTERVIEWED?

You will probably be interviewed and asked for references; you may be required to sign a form declaring that you do not have any health problems or a criminal record. You may also meet other volunteers in your area, who will explain the procedure for becoming a carer and what the work involves.

WHAT KIND OF WORK IS INVOLVED?

The type of work can vary from a couple of hours a day spent helping an elderly person with gardening, to sitting overnight with someone who is ill. You will never be expected to be involved in any task, or care for any person, if it makes you feel uncomfortable.

WHAT SKILLS DO I NEED?

You do not need any specialist skills to volunteer to be a carer. You should be offered training ranging from how to communicate with a wide variety of people, to basic first-aid and care skills. The skills gained as a volunteer will help you in all walks of life, and working in the community is widely respected by employers. The experience you gain may be accredited to other training schemes.

HOW MANY HOURS WILL I HAVE TO WORK?

The number of hours you agree to work is entirely up to you; you can arrange times to suit your lifestyle and other commitments. You can be flexible, but you must give notice if you cannot carry out your duties.

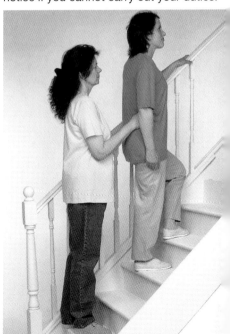

WORKING WITH PROFESSIONALS

You may be required to liaise with a number of professional people, such as Public Health Nurses and social workers. These people are responsible for assessing the level of care needed by the person you are caring for, and ensuring that it is carried out. When working with care professionals, you will be under their guidance, complementing, rather than replacing, their duties.

UNDERSTANDING YOUR ROLE

The care professional will delegate tasks to you or ask you to assist him. You may also be required to help a home carer so that he or she is able to have some time off.

BEING RELIABLE

Reliability is a key element in your relations with professional care workers/home carers. If you cannot meet a commitment, you should always try to give plenty of notice so that alternative arrangements can be made. If you cancel at the last minute, or fail to turn up at all, you will be letting down the person being cared for and may be compromising the good name of the voluntary organisation for which you work.

FOLLOWING A CARE PLAN

Your Public Health Nurse may give you a care plan that has been devised following an assessment of the person requiring care. If you are given such a plan, you should always adhere to the recommendations made in it.

The type of care
The requirements of the person being cared for and the kind of activities you will need to carry out.

The level of care
The extent and frequency of the care you will give to that person.

The objectives of the care
What specific aims the care plan is trying to achieve.

WHAT YOU CAN OFFER

You may see the person you are caring for more often than the care professional. If you notice improvements or a deterioration in the person's health, or recognise any deficiencies in the care plan, you should discuss these with the support services and Public Health Nurse.

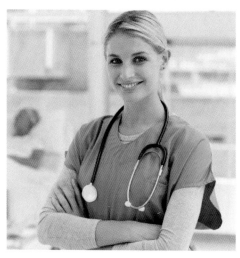

CARING FOR SOMEONE

Even though, as a volunteer carer, you are not a qualified professional, you should not think of yourself as an amateur. It is important that you act professionally so that the person you are caring for trusts you. Although you may become a close companion or a friend, you should still remember to behave responsibly and maintain confidentiality at all times.

SATISFY THE NEEDS OF THE CARED FOR

The most important aspect of your voluntary role is to provide care without depriving the person of her independence and self-confidence.

Individuality The person being cared for has needs and preferences that should be respected. Try to understand why she may be acting in a certain way.

Independence Wherever possible, allow the person to make decisions and do things for herself, even if this means that a task takes longer. Always ask her opinion and respect her views.

Confidence If the person being cared for feels she is a burden to everyone, she will become lonely and insecure. Comfort and reassure her, and encourage her to focus on the skills and abilities she still has.

BE AWARE OF YOUR OWN LIMITATIONS

As a volunteer you will be giving much of your time to others, and may be dealing with stressful situations. If you are dissatisfied or unhappy, it will be difficult for you to provide the best care.

Having limited skills You may feel that you have not been fully trained or are not qualified to deal with some of the tasks required of you, and that you are encroaching on the work of the care professional.

Feeling uncomfortable It may be that you don't get on with the person you are caring for, or feel ill at ease in the environment in which you are working.

Being unable to give enough You may feel that you are being asked to provide more care than you are able to offer. Try to recognise your own limitations and, if they affect the quality of the care you are providing, discuss them with your supervisor.

THE HOME CARER

As a volunteer carer, you may be in close contact with a home carer. Your relationship with that person is as important as your relationship with the person being cared for. It is essential that you work well as a team.

Practical support You can help with day-to-day tasks or provide night-time care so that the home carer has some time to themselves. You can also observe and ensure that the carer is aware and availing of all the resources and services available to them. The carer may value your help in obtaining advice and information.

Emotional support The home carer may lead an isolated life, and may find the burden of caring very arduous. Just being there to support and listen may help.

HOW A CARE PLAN CAN HELP YOU

When someone needs care, a plan is essential as it provides a clear breakdown of the person's requirements. It can be used by other volunteer carers or care professionals who come into the home. The plan should be provided by a care professional, who may ask you to help devise it or make recommendations. If, for any reason, it is not provided, request one from your supervisor or seek specific guidance about the type of care that the person requires. An example of a care plan is shown below.

CARE PLAN	NAME - MARY MURPHY* AGE - 91
ACTIVITY	**ASSESSMENT**
MOBILITY	Mobile with the use of a walking stick. A wheelchair should be used for long distances.
WASHING	Can wash unaided; needs help to get into and out of the bath.
DRESSING	Needs basic supervision.
EATING	Needs some help and encouragement. Prefers to eat with a spoon from a bowl, so cut food up or give soft foods if possible. Likes hot chocolate in the evening.
CONTINENCE	No problem.
SIGHT	Poor vision, even with spectacles.
HEARING	Adequate. Good with the use of an aid.
BEHAVIOUR	Mildly confused at times. Should be informed about any visitors.
MEDICATION	Twice daily for arthritis, with morning and evening meals.
COMMUNICATION	Mostly retains information and indicates needs verbally.
FINANCES	Managed by her daughter.
SOCIAL ACTIVITIES	Enjoys joining arranged activities. Attends day centre alternate weeks on a Wednesday.
HOBBIES	Enjoys listening to the radio and having the newspaper read to her.
LEVEL OF CARE	Mary needs care twice daily from Monday to Friday (her daughter cares for her at weekends). She should be visited first thing in the morning and in the afternoon. She receives Meals on Wheels at lunchtime, but her evening meal should be prepared for her.
OBJECTIVES OF CARE	Mary is quite able, and should be encouraged to be independent. Regular attendance at a day centre has been successful. Aim for attendance at least once a week by the end of the year.

Mary Murphy is not a real person

HOW TO TREAT THE CARED FOR

The way you treat the person you are caring for will affect how she feels about herself. It is important that you respect her needs and that she trusts you. If respect and trust are established early on, you should be able to form a mutually beneficial relationship.

RESPECT THE INDIVIDUAL

When caring for someone, treat her with the utmost respect. Ask yourself, 'How would I like to be treated?' and make this the basis for the standard of care that you want to achieve. Find out as much as you can about the person you are caring for, and respect her individual needs. She may, for example, have specific dietary needs, be of a different sexual orientation or different culture. Never forget that the person you are caring for is an individual in her own right, and is entitled to know what is happening to her. If there are changes to the care orders, take the time to explain them to her and, if possible, involve her in any decisions.

MAINTAIN CONFIDENTIALITY

It is important that the person you are caring for trusts you. To achieve this trust, you should respect her privacy and maintain confidentiality at all times. You have a duty to keep any information you may learn in your caring role absolutely confidential, including anything contained in the person's care records. The only exception to this is if you suspect abuse of any kind; report this to your GP, Public Health Nurse or supervisor immediately.

ADDRESSING PROBLEMS

You may not immediately feel at ease with the person you are caring for, but, over time, you may be able to develop a good relationship. In some circumstances, however, you may be completely incompatible with the person, to the point where you cannot carry out care duties effectively. If these differences cannot be resolved, ask to be removed from the duties. Remember, however, to strive for professionalism, even when you cannot communicate effectively with the person you are caring for.

SIGNS OF ABUSE

Abuse does occur and it could be the carer or the cared for who is the abuser. If you suspect abuse of any kind, inform your GP or Public Health Nurse.

Physical or sexual abuse Look out for physical signs such as negative body language.

Emotional abuse This might be one person shouting constantly at the other, belittling her or keeping her isolated. It may result in the victim of abuse being quiet and withdrawn.

Abuse by neglect Intentional or unintentional, refusal or failure to fulfil care giving obligation.

Financial abuse If you notice any financial irregularities, or stealing from the person you are caring for, inform your Public Health Nurse / supervisor. Keep receipts for goods that you buy on behalf of the person, so that your conduct is beyond reproach. (See page 36).

CHAPTER 3

COMMUNICATION

Talking and listening to one another are essential human needs. People need to communicate in order to express their anxieties and emotions, and to make their wishes known. Keeping the communication channels open when caring for your relative can be beneficial to both of you, and it is important to know what to do when this becomes difficult.

COMMUNICATION SKILLS

Most human beings take verbal communication for granted, so much so that they may, sometimes, not bother to make time for conversation. When you are caring for your relative, making the time to talk and listen can enhance your relationship and help to iron out any difficulties. You may be caring for someone with impaired senses, for whom verbal communication may be impossible; in such a situation you may need to rely on non-verbal skills, such as reading his body language and thinking about how you use your own. Do not, for example, be afraid to use touch, which can be reassuring as well as being an effective way of conveying your feelings. You will also need to explore ways to help your relative to improve his communication skills. This may be achieved by seeking specialist help and finding out if there are any aids available that cater for your relative's particular needs.

TALKING AND LISTENING

Finding time for conversation is very important, especially to someone who is housebound or does not have contact with many people. It is easy to find excuses not to talk or listen, but if you make the time you may feel closer to the person you are caring for. Proper communication will allow both of you to express your feelings and help to prevent resentment building up.

IMPROVING COMMUNICATION

There are many reasons why communication can break down, making it difficult for you and your relative to talk to each other. It is important to keep the lines of communication open and address any problems as early as possible.

MAKE TIME TO TALK

If you and your relative spend long periods of time together, you may become so familiar with each other that you do not notice hours passing without conversation. Also, as a carer, you will undoubtedly be extremely busy, and it may seem like a luxury to sit down and talk. But try not to think of it like that; allocate time to talk, even if it is only over a cup of tea or between television programmes. It could mean a lot to your relative.

FIND COMMON INTERESTS

If your own lifestyle is restricted, it may be difficult to find things to talk about. However, it is usually possible to find subjects of mutual interest, such as sport, gardening or television. Do not be afraid to talk about yourself and your interests. If your friends visit, try to include your relative in the discussions.

BE PATIENT

If your relative suffers from confusion or has impaired speech or hearing, verbal communication can be difficult and frustrating. You may sometimes feel that your patience is being pushed to the limit. Instead of getting angry, try taking deep breaths to calm yourself down or, after ensuring that your relative is safe, leave the room for a few minutes until you are feeling less wound up.

DO'S & DON'TS

- **Do** try to think about the way you are speaking and how your voice sounds. The pitch, rate and rhythm of your voice are important if your relative has impaired hearing.
- **Do** be patient if your relative has impaired speech. Give him time to finish his sentence and resist the temptation to interrupt or speak for him.
- **Don't** patronise your relative. Whatever his disability, he should be treated with respect and not be addressed as if he were a child. A person who is physically impaired is still likely to be mentally alert.
- **Don't** exclude your relative from group conversations, whatever his condition. It may make him feel isolated and worthless if he is left alone in a corner watching and listening to other people talking.

A VOLUNTEER CARER

When you are a carer from outside the home, it is essential to communicate effectively with the person you are looking after and the home carer, if there is one. This may range from the simple matter of addressing someone appropriately, to overcoming language or cultural differences. Finding out as much as possible about the person you are caring for will help.

LANGUAGE AND CULTURAL DIFFERENCES

If the person you are caring for speaks a different language, communication can be difficult, but over time it should become easier. Be aware of any different cultural beliefs, and respect the fact that he may want to do things in a different way.

USE AN INTERPRETER

You may find that younger members of the family speak fluent English. Communicate either through one of them or ask your supervisor to arrange for an interpreter to accompany you, at least initially.

EDUCATE YOURSELF

Find out as much as possible about the person's beliefs by speaking to him or his family, and by obtaining information from your supervisor or local authority.

RESPECT THE PERSON'S WISHES

Beliefs and traditions may affect someone's lifestyle; this could include dietary restrictions or a woman not being allowed to be seen by a male doctor.

BE AWARE OF ISOLATION

Some members of ethnic minorities may have no contacts outside their immediate family, which may lead to a feeling of isolation. Discuss this problem with the affected person and his family, and try to find local activities that enable him to meet people who share his beliefs and interests.

RELATING TO THE HOME CARER

If there is already a carer in the home, he or she may resent your presence or even see it as an intrusion. Reassure him or her that you are there to support and not to take over and work to identify ways in which you can help.

Advice and support
You may be able to help with practical problems and, if he or she asks for it, give advice on the benefits and resources that are available.

Companionship The home carer may not come into contact with many people; he or she may welcome a friendly face and the chance to talk to someone else.

Level of care If you and the home carer communicate well with each other and work together, the overall level of care given should improve, which will be beneficial to the person being cared for.

USING BODY LANGUAGE

Although most of us express ourselves through the spoken word, we also communicate in many non-verbal ways. When you are caring for your relative, it can help if you understand his body language and know how to use your own. Body language is even more important if your relative's speech and hearing are impaired, rendering him unable to communicate verbally.

SIGNS OF ABUSE

You may suspect from your relative's body language that he is the victim of physical, sexual or emotional abuse. Abuse can take place in the home, as well as when the person is being cared for elsewhere. If you suspect abuse of any kind, alert a GP or Public Health Nurse. Look out for behavioural changes or signs of injury.

Withdrawal

The abused may isolate himself. He may appear wary of people and withdraw when he is approached.

Depression

The person may appear depressed or unusually quiet and avoid communication, especially eye contact.

Injury

The abused may try to cover up bruising or other injuries. He may give unlikely explanations for how he has sustained his injuries. (See page 32)

THE PERSON BEING CARED FOR

Learning to read body language will help you to care more effectively for your relative.

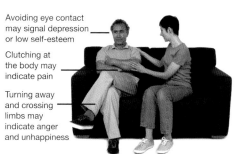

Avoiding eye contact may signal depression or low self-esteem

Clutching at the body may indicate pain

Turning away and crossing limbs may indicate anger and unhappiness

THE CARER

You can use your body language to help your relative feel more secure and so improve communication.

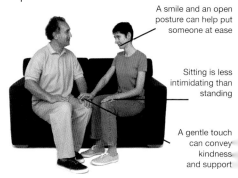

A smile and an open posture can help put someone at ease

Sitting is less intimidating than standing

A gentle touch can convey kindness and support

ADAPTING FOR SPECIAL NEEDS

Communication difficulties may arise when you are caring for someone with impaired speech, sight or hearing. It is possible to overcome these difficulties by adapting the way in which you communicate. Many aids are available to help someone who has impaired senses to improve his ability to communicate and encourage independence.

IMPAIRED SPEECH

Helping someone to relearn how to speak can take a long time, and requires a great deal of perseverance, patience and encouragement. Talk to your relative's GP or Public Health Nurse to find out what specialist help is available.

REASONS FOR SPEECH LOSS

There are different reasons for speech loss or impairment of the voice.

Stroke The loss of speech that can occur after a stroke will be sudden. Your relative may know what he wants, but be unable to communicate his needs, which can be very distressing. Often, he will literally have to be taught to speak again.

Voice box removal Someone who has had his voice box (larynx) removed will be more prepared for loss of speech. He may have a special device fitted that enables him to speak by modifying the sound produced by belching air from his stomach. This relearning process takes time and requires patience.

Brain damage Someone who is brain-damaged may be able to speak, but be unable to find the right word. This can be frustrating for both of you, but with patience you can learn to understand his needs.

GETTING SPECIALIST HELP

You may, in time, learn to recognise what your relative is trying to say, but it will help both of you if you seek the help of a specialist.

Ask to see a speech therapist A GP can refer your relative to a speech therapist, who is trained to recognise the nature of speech problems and how to overcome them. With his guidance, you will be able to help your relative with exercises, such as how to shape the mouth to form different sounds.

COMMUNICATION AIDS

A person with impaired speech will be helped by having one or more of the items below to hand.

Pencil and paper These should always be close to hand, so that your relative can write down requests.

Mechanical aids Specialist machines are available for your relative to communicate their needs i.e. computers.

Visual aids Can be used to identify frequently used items.

Pictures Stick images from magazines on to cards.

IMPAIRED SIGHT

This may be a condition present since birth, or it may come about as the result of disease or injury. If your relative's loss of sight is sudden, due, say, to an accident, it may be very frightening for him. If it develops gradually, you will both have time to get used to it and make the necessary adjustments. Where possible, try to help your relative to maintain independence.

TYPES OF SIGHT LOSS

The level of impairment varies from person to person; few people have a complete lack of vision. Understanding the type of sight loss can enable you to help your relative. For instance, he may:

- distinguish only light;
- have no central vision;
- have no side vision;
- see only a vague blur;
- see only a mixture of blank spaces and defined areas.

COMMUNICATING WITH EACH OTHER

It is essential that your relative is independent and feels at ease in his home. The way you communicate with him is very important and may require you to adapt the way you would normally speak or respond.

Non-verbal signs Avoid responding non-verbally, by nodding or shaking your head. Also, remember that body language, such as a smile or an outstretched hand, may be impossible for your relative to see.

Greetings and farewells When you approach a blind person, always say 'Hello' and take his hand to shake it or pat his arm or shoulder to reassure him. If you do not know him well, identify yourself. Tell him when you are leaving, so that he is not left talking to himself.

Talking Do not change the way you speak. Do not be afraid to say 'Nice to see you' - most blind people use this phrase themselves. If you and the person are in company, address him by name or use a light touch on the arm to indicate that you are speaking to him.

Personal space To allow your relative maximum independence in the home, make sure his belongings and the items he frequently uses are kept in the same place; this will make it easier for him to locate things.

INDEPENDENCE AIDS

Being registered blind (by an ophthalmologist) may provide entitlement to a range of special services, allowances and equipment.

Telling the time
Clocks and watches with raised dots allow the person to tell the time.

Playing games
Modified sets of popular games are available

Reading and writing
Braille is a system of printing in raised dots that can be read by touch. 'Talking' books and large-print text also provide access to books.

Writing aid
This enables a visually impaired person to write in straight lines.

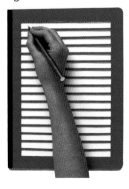

IMPAIRED HEARING

It is quite common for an elderly person's hearing to fail gradually. He may not realise that he is becoming deaf, or he may even refuse to accept his condition. Deafness may lead to feelings of isolation and rejection, and the person may think that people are talking about him or laughing at him behind his back. Try to be patient and reassuring.

COMMUNICATING WITH EACH OTHER

By reassessing the way in which you speak and the implications of your body language, you should be able to overcome the difficulties involved in communicating effectively.

Facing someone When you are talking to someone with impaired hearing, always face him so that he can lip-read what you are saying.

Tone of voice Learn to use the lower tones of your voice range, as someone with impaired hearing is more able to hear these.

Body language Use non-verbal communication as much as possible. Your body language may be an essential way of communicating with someone with impaired hearing.

Sign language If your relative is deaf, it is useful to learn sign language. You could also develop your own signs between you.

INDEPENDENCE AIDS

There is a range of aids available to help those with impaired hearing.

Hearing aid

In order to ensure the hearing aid fits properly, a mould of your relative's ear will be taken. He should be warned that a hearing aid will magnify all sounds equally, so that he is prepared for this when he is in particularly noisy places. In order to work effectively, the hearing aid should not be allowed to get wet, and the batteries should be checked regularly.

Specialist telephones

A variety of telephones are available; a flashing light can indicate ringing and some display the message on a screen.

Amplifying sound

Personal amplifiers increase the sound of a radio or television. Portable amplifiers that attach to the earpiece of a telephone are also available.

Facing person allows him to lip-read

Sign language facilitates communication

DEALING WITH CONFUSION

If a person is confused, he may forget simple facts, such as what day of the week it is, who someone is or his whereabouts. This can be frustrating for both of you and potentially dangerous for your relative. Although looking after a confused person requires patience, there are practical steps you can take to help him to remember things and become less dependent on you.

MEMORY LOSS

Confusion can cause or be the result of memory loss. Someone who has lost the ability to add to his long-term memory may forget something you said ten seconds ago, but be able to remember clearly an event that happened ten years ago. He may ask you the same question over and over again; not only has he forgotten the answer, he has probably forgotten that he ever asked you the question.

COMMUNICATING INFORMATION

You can help your relative by thinking about the way you communicate information.
Use active phrases Say, 'It is time to take your tablets'. Do not tell him hours before, 'You need to take your tablets at three o'clock'.
Be specific Be precise when writing a reminder: 'Your hospital appointment is at 11am on Thursday, 16th May', not 'Hospital appointment, Thursday'.
Keep questions direct Ask your relative, 'Would you like tea or coffee?' Do not ask him, 'What would you like to drink?'

INDEPENDENCE AIDS

Use some of the methods recommended below to encourage independence. Discuss these with your relative first, as he may resent the house being cluttered with reminders telling him what to do. **Clocks and calendars** All clocks and calendars should be correct; an alarm clock could be set to ring at the time your relative requires his medication. **Notice board** List the things that are happening that day, such as visitors expected or outings planned. **Notes** Place reminder notes, such as 'Have you turned the oven off?' strategically.

SHORT-TERM CONFUSION

Confusion is not always a long-term problem. Quite often, it can be a temporary condition that is most common when the person is ill.
Due to illness
Sometimes an acute infection, for instance, can cause temporary confusion. You should give your relative plenty of fluids to prevent him from becoming dehydrated and help lessen the confusion. Consult the GP or Public Health Nurse for advice.
Drug-related
Confusion and behavioural changes may coincide with your relative being put on new medication. If this occurs, inform the GP of the problem so that a change of medication or dosage can be considered. Drug-related confusion can also occur when a person has been on long-term medication.

CHAPTER 4

ADAPTING THE HOME

One of the main aims of caring is to help your relative to maintain independence. To achieve this, it may be necessary to make some changes to the home environment. Always seek the advice of an occupational therapist before embarking on any adaptations or purchasing specialist equipment. An occupational therapist is trained to assess the needs of the person you are caring for and advise on possible funding.

WHAT YOU CAN DO

Adaptations should always be safe and, wherever possible, also suitable for able-bodied members of the household. Simple measures, such as rearranging furniture and moving unnecessary clutter out of the way, can create space and allow someone to move around more easily; giving thought to where frequently needed items are placed can enable your relative to do more for herself. If she has mobility problems or is a wheelchair user, it may be necessary to obtain specialist equipment or make structural changes, such as widening doors. It is essential that you discuss any changes with your relative beforehand and that she is happy with them, otherwise it could be confusing for her to find things rearranged, especially if she has been in hospital for some time.

THE PATIENT'S SURROUNDINGS

The majority of people are usually able to choose their environment. If anything makes it uncomfortable or dangerous, they are free to make adjustments or move away. Persons confined to bed are dependent upon those nursing them to see that their surroundings are safe.

THE PATIENT'S ROOM

A room on the ground floor would be ideal with easy access to the bathroom and toilet facilities and a window looking out onto a garden. It should be cheerful yet restful with adequate space, heating, lighting and ventilation without a draft. Basic essential furniture is needed to suit the requirements and needs of the patient, for example, a radio, television and a reading light. The room should be accessible and easy to clean. Damp dusting is recommended and the use of mats avoided. Flowers and fruit should be removed overnight. One or two visitors at a time is preferable as too many may be over-powering. Everything must be done to provide a safe and comfortable environment for both carer and patient. A good atmosphere will have a positive effect on the patient.

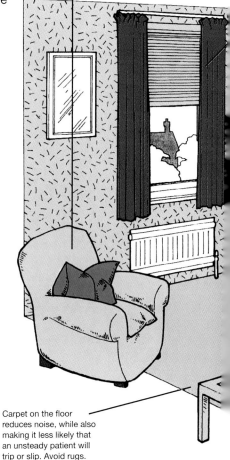

A comfortable armchair should provide good support for the patient's back when he is relaxing out of bed.

Carpet on the floor reduces noise, while also making it less likely that an unsteady patient will trip or slip. Avoid rugs.

A good-sized table becomes a surface on which to lay out equipment before treatment.

A bedside cupboard provides the patient with a convenient surface for everything he needs to have within reach, as well as storage space. Provide a good bedside light and a handbell.

The ideal bed in which to nurse the patient is a single bed with access on three sides and a clear path between the bed and the door.

Curtains are most efficient for excluding draughts.

A bed-tray is invaluable for the patient who has to have his meals in bed.

Two upright chairs are needed for visitors and for bedmaking.

A commode of the type that doubles as an ordinary chair is useful for patients who cannot get as far as the bathroom.

PROMOTING SAFETY AND INDEPENDENCE IN THE HOME

Doing things differently in the home and the use of special equipment may make caring for a person easier. The person you are caring for may need to be encouraged to do as much as they can for themselves.

A variety of aids and appliances are available to assist people with daily living activities. A public health nurse, occupational therapist or physiotherapist will advise and assess your needs, and subject to financial eligibility, can order appropriate equipment or advise on where they can be purchased.

- Do not let strangers into your house
- Phone the Gardaí if you are worried/suspicious

SAFETY AND SECURITY TIPS

- Wear a personal alarm and ensure it is on
- Have emergency telephone numbers in large writing
- Leave a spare key with a friend or neighbour
- Have a safety chain, spy hole and intercom fitted on your front door
- Ensure smoke detectors are installed and working
- Keep a fire extinguisher and fire blanket in the kitchen
- Place an effective spark guard in front of open fire
- Report smells of gas to the Gas Company
- Don't overload electric sockets and have electric equipment checked regularly
- Have a night-light
- Do not smoke in bed, it can be fatal

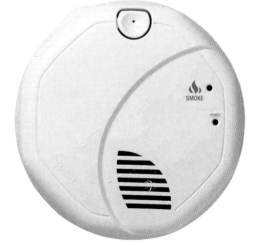

Smoke Detector

CHAPTER 5

HOME HYGIENE

If your relative is ill or frail, or is taking certain medication, he may be particularly vulnerable to infection, so it is essential to maintain as hygienic and germ-free an environment as possible. It is also important to protect yourself from infection, because if you become ill, not only will you be unable to fulfil your role efficiently, you may also put the health of your relative at risk.

CLEANLINESS
There are many preventive measures you can take to eliminate germs (bacteria and viruses) and minimise the spread of infection. The most important of these measures is to maintain a high standard of personal hygiene: a simple task such as hand washing is often done in a quick, perfunctory way, but washing your hands thoroughly is an essential part of basic cleanliness.

DISPOSAL OF WASTE
If your relative is ill or incontinent, part of your caring role may include dealing with the disposal of his body waste, such as blood, faeces, vomit or urine. It is essential that you follow the correct procedures for the disposal of this waste to minimise the risk of infecting yourself, and to prevent any infection from spreading to other people.

INFECTION AND ITS CAUSES

An infection is the result of the body being invaded by germs (bacteria and viruses). This causes an adverse reaction - directly by damaging cells, or indirectly by releasing poisonous substances (toxins) into the body. The symptoms will depend on the type of infection, where it is located and whether it has spread throughout the body.

HOW INFECTION SPREADS

Anyone can become infected, but the most vulnerable are those who have not been vaccinated, and those who have low immunity, such as a frail person or someone in poor health. An infection is only dangerous if it is given a suitable environment in which to flourish.

Sources People and animals are the sources of most infections, carrying many bacteria and viruses.

Routes An infection can be passed on through direct and indirect routes (see below).

DIRECT AND INDIRECT ROUTES

A person can catch an infection directly by touching something that is contaminated; by sharing a needle with a contaminated person; through an exchange of body fluids such as blood or saliva; or through sexual activity with an infected person. An infection can be spread indirectly in a variety of ways.

Airborne Germs can be carried in the droplets of fluid expelled when coughing and sneezing.

Food This can become contaminated if it is not stored, handled or cooked correctly.

Clothing or equipment These can harbour germs if they are not cleaned regularly and thoroughly.

Insects A number of insects, especially house flies, can spread infection.

TREATING INFECTION

If you suspect that you or your relative has an infection, seek medical help as soon as possible. The GP may prescribe a course of antibiotics for bacterial infections; these will only be effective if the course is completed. If the infection is viral, the GP will usually only be able to treat the symptoms while the immune system clears the virus.

THE SYMPTOMS OF INFECTION

The symptoms of an infection depend on whether the infection is confined to one area or has spread throughout the body. For example, an infection caused by an abscess may be localised, whereas the nfection caused by chickenpox, measles or a common cold will affect the whole body. Symptoms of a localised infection may be:
- pain and swelling;
- localised redness;
- loss of movement;
- areas that are hot to the touch.

Symptoms of an infection throughout the body may be:
- high temperature and increased breathing and pulse rates;
- headache and thirst;
- hot, dry skin and rash;
- loss of appetite;
- weakness and apathy.

DISPOSING OF BODY WASTE

When you are caring for someone, you should take precautions to prevent yourself, and anyone else, from coming into contact with that person's body waste. The risk of spreading infection can be greatly reduced if you take the necessary preventive measures. When disposing of waste, wear latex gloves and an apron, if available. If you are caring for someone who is known to be suffering from a blood-borne infection, such as HIV or hepatitis, seek advice from the person's GP.

METHODS OF DISPOSAL

There are two safe ways to dispose of waste.

Down the toilet Place body fluids and soiled tissues in the toilet bowl, close the lid and flush the toilet twice.

In a plastic bag Some waste materials, such as dressings and incontinence pads, should be placed in a secure plastic bag, which must be sealed before being placed in the rubbish bin - never flush them down the toilet. If your relative has a blood-borne infection, official yellow plastic bags will be supplied and collected for incineration.

CLEANING SPILLAGES

Wearing latex gloves, cover the body waste with paper towels and pour household cleaning agent over the towels if the waste is on a hard surface. It can then be collected and disposed of in a sealed plastic bag. If the spill is on a carpet, use hot, soapy water, not bleach.

NEEDLESTICK INJURY

If you accidentally prick yourself with a used needle, or other sharp object that has come into contact with body fluids, do not suck the injury or stop it from bleeding. To prevent the spread of infection, follow this procedure:

- wash the affected area under cold, running water;
- encourage the wound to bleed freely;
- attend an A&E Department where a protocol will be in place to manage such an incident

If you are a volunteer carer, you must inform the organisation for whom you are working so that the incident can be documented.

NEEDLE AND SYRINGE DISPOSAL

If a medication has to be given by injection, or your relative has to test his blood through pin-pricks, the safe disposal of needles and syringes is essential. These should be placed in a special approved container, called a 'sharps' box, which is supplied by local health services, but is also available from chemists. A healthcare professional will arrange to collect and dispose of the box at regular agreed intervals.

Follow these guidelines:

- keep the sharps box out of the reach of children as they may be able to access the needles;
- do not fill the box beyond the three quarters level;
- do not place the box in a domestic bin-bag.

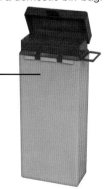

Sharps box

Special container for safe needle and syringe disposal

SOME INFECTIOUS DISEASES

DISEASE	POSSIBLE SIGNS AND SYMPTOMS	HOW IT MAY BE TRANSMITTED	INFECTIOUS PERIOD
CHICKENPOX	Slight fever, groups of itchy, red spots that become blisters.	Airborne. Contact with rash.	Until all blisters crust over.
GASTROENTERITIS	Appetite loss, nausea, vomiting, diarrhoea, abdominal cramps.	Contaminated food or water supplies.	Up to 2 days after diarrhoea stops.
GLANDULAR FEVER	Fever, headache, swollen glands in neck, armpits and groin, severe sore throat, fatigue.	Contact with saliva.	Variable - may be weeks.
HEPATITIS A, B, C, D AND E	Flu-like illness followed by jaundice. Some people have no symptoms.	A, E: infected food or water. B, C, D: sexually transmitted; contaminated blood; shared needles.	A, E: one week after jaundice. B, C, D: varies; blood can be infectious for life.
HERPES SIMPLEX (COLD SORES & GENITAL HERPES)	Small, fluid-filled, irritating blisters, slight temperature.	Contact with lesions.	Until blisters crust over.
HIV/AIDS	May be symptomless for years; breathlessness, fever, weight loss, diarrhoea, swollen glands and fatigue may eventually occur.	Sexually transmitted; contaminated blood; shared needles; mother to child in utero.	For life.
INFLUENZA, COMMON COLD	Fever, cough, runny nose, headache, sore throat, chills, aches, pains.	Airborne.	First few days.

SOME INFECTIOUS DISEASES (CONT...)

DISEASE	POSSIBLE SIGNS AND SYMPTOMS	HOW IT MAY BE TRANSMITTED	INFECTIOUS PERIOD
MEASLES	Raised temperature, watery eyes and nose; light pink rash.	Droplet/Airborne.	From onset of symptoms to 4 days after onset of rash.
MENINGITIS	Fever, headache, drowsiness, confusion, rash, reaction to light.	Various methods, usually airborne.	Will depend on the causative organism.
MUMPS	Viral infection causing swelling in salivary glands in the face principally in front of the ears.	Droplet/Airborne.	3 days before salivary swelling to 4 days after.
RUBELLA OR (GERMAN MEASLES)	Light pink rash.	Droplet/Airborne.	7 days before onset of rash to 4 days after.
SHINGLES	Localised, painful blistering rash.	Reactivation of chickenpox virus present in the body.	Not infectious.
TUBERCULOSIS	Fever, cough, swollen and painful glands, stiff neck, weight loss.	Airborne.	While phlegm is infected.
WHOOPING COUGH	Severe bouts of coughing followed by an inspiratory whooping noise and often vomiting.	Airborne.	7 days after exposure to 3 weeks after onset of symptoms (shortened to 1 week with antibiotic use).

Vaccinations are essential to avoid certain infectious diseases. It is important to keep up to date with health services guidelines.

PREVENTING INFECTION

The body's immune system cannot fully protect against infection. It is essential, therefore, for your own health and that of your relative, to take steps to eliminate the germs that cause infection from your home environment. The risks can be minimised if you maintain a good level of cleanliness and take proper precautions when dealing with body waste.

PERSONAL HYGIENE

You can maintain a high standard of cleanliness, and minimise the risk of infection, by washing your hands thoroughly and wearing disposable gloves. It is important that you follow the correct technique for removing gloves once they are soiled.

WASHING YOUR HANDS THOROUGHLY

Wash your hands before and after preparing food, after using the toilet and before and after giving care, even if gloves are worn. Scrub dirty nails as part of your hand washing routine.

1 Wet and soap your hands. Rub your palms together to form a lather.

To clean thoroughly, build up rich lather

2 Rub the palm and fingers of one hand over the back of the other, interlocking the fingers. Repeat for the other hand.

Clean back of hand and between fingers

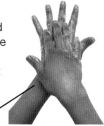

THE BODY'S NATURAL DEFENCES

The immune system is the body's main defence against infection. White blood cells circulate around the body and destroy harmful bacteria. People on chemotherapy, for example, who have a low number of these cells, will be more prone to infection.

Clean palms and backs of fingers simultaneously

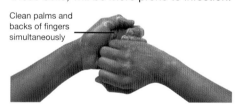

3 Lock together the closed fingers of both hands and rub the backs of them against your palms.

Clean thumbs and fronts of fingers simultaneously

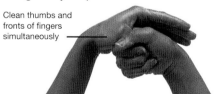

4 Clean each thumb by rubbing it against the insides of your fingers.

5 Clean your fingertips by rubbing them on the palm of the opposite hand. This also cleans the palm.

6 Rinse your hands and dry them on a clean cloth or paper towel.

WEARING AND REMOVING GLOVES

Gloves should be worn whenever a procedure involves contact with body fluids, and when creams or lotions are being applied. To prevent any substance coming into contact with your skin, always remove gloves following the procedure below. Disposable latex or vinyl gloves are available from most chemists. The thinner, polythene varieties should not be used as they do not provide adequate protection.

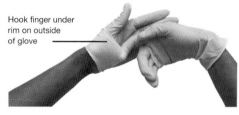

Hook finger under rim on outside of glove

1 Pick up the base of the left-hand glove with your right index finger. Pull it halfway off your hand, leaving the top half of your thumb covered.

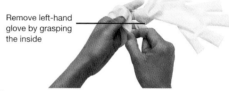

Keep left-hand glove half on

Grip right hand glove under rim

2 Repeat step 1 to remove the glove on your right hand, but this time pull the glove all the way off, so that it is completely inside out.

Remove left-hand glove by grasping the inside

3 Use your now uncovered right hand to pull the left glove off, so that both gloves are now inside out.

4 Pick up the gloves on the inside, dispose of them safely and wash your hands thoroughly.

CLEANING EQUIPMENT

Some of the items used when caring may be disposable, but others will require thorough cleaning. Always wear gloves.

Toilet aids Clean bedpans, urinals and commode pans with hot, soapy water.

Washing accessories Wash flannels and towels regularly. It is advisable to use separate towels and flannels on the face and body.

Surfaces Clean surfaces such as table-tops and bed-trays with a detergent, and dry thoroughly with a clean cloth.

CONTAINING YOUR OWN GERMS

It is particularly important to take steps to ensure that you do not spread your own germs to your relative.

Illness If you are ill, it will not be beneficial to you or your relative if you continue caring. Inform a care professional so that alternative arrangements can be made.

Coughing and sneezing Use a tissue or handkerchief and avoid coughing or sneezing in the direction of your relative.

Skin infections If you have cuts, abrasions or a skin disorder, you must ensure that the entire area is properly protected by gloves or a waterproof dressing before giving care.

WHAT ELSE MUST BE CONSIDERED?

- Keep items such as toothbrushes, sponges, face cloths and towels for the person you are caring for separate. Colour coding can be an effective way to achieve this. This will reduce the risk of infection spreading to other members of the family;
- If you suspect the person has an infection, wear disposable gloves;
- When cleaning spillages, wear disposable gloves, gather it all up with clean paper towels and dispose of it in a sealed plastic bag.

KITCHEN

It is essential to take simple steps when preparing and cooking food to reduce the risk of contamination. In order to minimise any health risks, you need to keep your kitchen and cooking utensils clean, shop sensibly, store food wisely and prepare it carefully.

HYGIENE TIPS

To prevent food contamination make the following simple steps part of your daily routine when using your kitchen.
- Wash your hands before and after preparing food;
- Clean utensils and cutting tools thoroughly;
- Change and wash cloths and towels regularly;
- Avoid wiping your hands repeatedly on an apron or cloth; do not use tea towels as hand towels;
- Cover any cuts or sores on your hands;
- Keep pets away from all food and kitchen surfaces.

PREPARING FOOD

- Do not eat food from damaged containers, or food that has passed its expiry date;
- Wash fresh fruit and vegetables thoroughly;
- Do not use the same knife or chopping board to prepare cooked and uncooked foods at the same time;
- Ensure raw and cooked/ready to eat foods are kept separately at all times;
- Do not prepare food too far in advance;
- Follow frozen food guidelines carefully;
- All food preparation surfaces and utensils should be thoroughly cleaned after use.

CHAPTER 6

HEALTHY EATING & DRINKING

Your relative may have a small appetite or find eating difficult because of an illness, a disability or general apathy, but it is essential that she is encouraged to eat well and regularly. Achieving a balanced diet is always possible, even if someone has to follow a special diet for health or personal reasons. To help you to meet the requirements of a balanced diet, this chapter provides a basic understanding of nutrition.

MAKING MEALTIMES ENJOYABLE

To make mealtimes enjoyable and relaxed, try to gain an understanding of your relative's needs and, if she is physically impaired, find practical ways that allow her to be more independent when eating or drinking. Simple measures can be taken to make meals look and taste as appetising as possible; this is especially important for someone who is ill and does not have a strong appetite.

CARING FOR YOURSELF

As a carer it is easy to neglect your own needs and get into bad habits, such as skipping meals or snacking. To meet the high energy demands required for caring, however, it is essential that you also eat sensibly and regularly.

GOLDEN RULES OF FOOD SAFETY

FOOD SAFETY TIPS

- Always cook food thoroughly, ensure meat juices run clear;
- When using a microwave always rotate and stir food and leave the cooked food standing for the recommended time;
- Use clean water from a mains supply;
- Once thawed, cook food immediately. Remember not to re-freeze thawed food in an uncooked state;
- Don't forget to re-heat cooked food thoroughly;
- Store food as directed on the label;
- Avoid contact between raw and cooked food. Always use separate cutting boards and utensils for cooked and raw food. This will prevent bacteria from a meat or poultry product contaminating another food. Otherwise, wash and disinfect between uses;
- Frequently wash your hands;
- Ensure kitchen surfaces are clean;
- Take care that food is stored at the correct temperature;
- Food should be protected from insects, rodents and pets;
- Transport chilled and frozen foods as quickly as possible to their final destination.

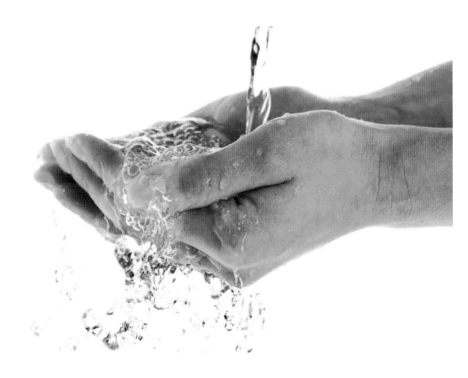

EATING A BALANCED DIET

To maintain good health you need to eat the right balance of foods from each of the five main food groups, and drink plenty of fluids. Provided no particular food is eaten to excess, and sufficient calories are consumed for the body's daily needs, your diet should be well balanced.

WHAT YOUR BODY NEEDS

Your body needs a combination of nutrients - proteins, carbohydrates, fats, vitamins, minerals and fibre - to satisfy all its requirements.

PROTEINS

Proteins supply the body with the amino acids that are required to build new protein. Animal foods provide all the essential amino acids, while plant foods need to be combined.

CARBOHYDRATES

These are starches or sugars and are the body's main source of energy. Starches are broken down into single molecules by the digestive system before being absorbed into the bloodstream, and often contain beneficial fibre. Sugars are absorbed rapidly, supplying an instant, but short-term, surge of energy.

FATS

These are a good energy source (especially for those who have high energy requirements, such as the elderly) and are an essential component of the body's cells. However, saturated fat in particular should be eaten in moderation, due to the risk of heart disease and obesity.

VITAMINS AND MINERALS

These are an essential part of a balanced diet; they help the body to function properly and contribute to overall good health.

FIBRE

This passes through the body unchanged and is essential in preventing bowel and digestive problems. Fibre is also filling and may, therefore, reduce calorie intake.

FOLIC ACID

Taking a folic acid tablet before becoming pregnant and during early pregnancy can reduce the risk of your baby being affected by neural tube defects such as spina bifida. Women who are planning to have a baby are advised to take one folic acid tablet daily before they conceive and for the first 12 weeks of pregnancy.

WHAT VITAMINS CAN DO

VITAMIN	WHAT IT DOES	WHERE IT CAN BE FOUND
A	Enhances normal growth, night vision, protects against infection.	Liver, fish-liver oils, egg yolk, dairy products, margarine, tomatoes, carrots.
VITAMIN B COMPLEX, INCLUDING B1, B2, B6	Helps the body to convert food into energy. Needed for growth and immune function.	Breads, cereals, meat, eggs, nuts and beans.
B12	Helps to form red blood cells and to keep the nervous system healthy.	Meat and meat products, chicken, fish, eggs, milk and dairy products.
C	Maintains healthy bones and teeth; aids iron absorption.	Vegetables, fruit, especially citrus fruit, potatoes.
D	Essential for strong bones and teeth; helps calcium absorption.	Oily fish, liver, milk, egg yolk, some spreads and margarine; made in skin from sunlight.
E	Aids formation of red blood cells; slows down cell ageing.	Vegetable oils, nuts, meat, green vegetables, cereals.
K	Promotes blood clotting.	Green vegetables and cereals. Made in the human intestine by bacteria.

WHAT MINERALS CAN DO

MINERAL	WHAT IT DOES	WHERE IT CAN BE FOUND
SODIUM	Helps regulate blood pressure. Needed for muscles & nerves to function.	Salt, bread, cereals, bacon, ham. Occurs naturally in most foods.
POTASSIUM	Regulates the heart; helps the function of the nervous system and kidneys; has many functions.	Meat, fish, fruit, vegetables.
CALCIUM	Keeps bones and teeth healthy. Also needed for healthy blood, nerves & muscles.	Milk, cheese, yoghurt, green leafy vegetables and beans.
IRON	A constituent of the oxygen carrying pigment of red blood cells.	Liver, meat, egg yolk, nuts, beans & fortified breakfast cereals.
FLUORIDE	Helps to harden the teeth and strengthen the bones.	Fish, tea, coffee, soya beans & fluoridated water.
IODINE	Aids action of thyroid gland, which controls growth and development.	Milk & seafood.

EATING FROM THE FIVE MAIN FOOD GROUPS

To maintain a balanced diet, you need to choose a combination of foods from the five main food groups. The chart below is a guide to the types of food in each group and the nutrients they provide. It also includes the recommended guidelines for what you should eat daily and gives tips on how to increase or decrease your intake of particular types of foods.

THE MAIN FOOD GROUPS

FOOD GROUP	WHAT IT CONTAINS	DAILY NEEDS
CEREALS & POTATOES	**Bread, pasta, oats, cereal, potatoes and rice** Good sources of starch and energy; rich in fibre, vitamins and minerals.	**Four portions** Boost your intake by eating all types, and opt for high fibre varieties where possible. Try not to eat them with added fat.
FRUIT & VEGETABLES	**Fruit and vegetables** These are a good source of vitamins, minerals and fibre. Fresh is best, but frozen, dried and tinned can also be eaten.	**Five or six portions** Eat some fruit and vegetables raw. A glass of fruit juice is one serving. Check tinned products for added salt or sugar.
MEAT, FISH & ALTERNATIVES	**Fish, nuts, meat, eggs, poultry, soya and seeds** These foods are good sources of protein, vitamins and minerals.	**Two portions** Choose lean cuts of meat, and fish such as salmon and herring. Remove the skin from poultry to reduce the fat content.
MILK & DAIRY PRODUCTS	**Cheese, yogurt and cream** Good sources of calcium and protein, but many products from this group have a high saturated fat content.	**Two portions** Choose low-fat varieties, such as semi-skimmed milk, low-fat yogurt and cheeses such as Edam.
FATTY & SUGARY FOODS	**Jam, butter, sweets, chocolate, oil, sugar and crisps** These are high in calories and provide the body with energy, but many contain saturated fats.	**Eat only occasionally** This is the only group that should not be eaten every day. Only eat these foods in small quantities. Try snacking on fruit and vegetables instead.

SPECIAL DIETS

You may have to adapt your relative's diet for health reasons or to satisfy her personal tastes. Always follow the advice of a nutritionist or doctor if your relative's diet is restricted for medical reasons, and respect your relative's wishes if she chooses not to eat certain foods. Whatever types of food you are providing, try to meet the requirements of a balanced diet.

A DIET FOR HEALTH REASONS

Certain illnesses and conditions can result in dietary restrictions. For example, someone with heart disease may have to reduce salt or fat intake, and a condition such as diabetes may necessitate a controlled sugar intake. A GP or nutritionist will be able to advise on what can and cannot be eaten.

A VEGETARIAN DIET

Vegetarians do not eat meat or fish. Most will eat some animal foods, such as dairy produce, but always check the person's preference. A vegetarian diet differs from a non-vegetarian one in several ways.

A low level of saturated fat Because of the absence of red meat in a vegetarian diet, the level of saturated fat content will be low.

A high level of fibre The diet is more likely to contain meat alternatives, such as beans, pulses and grains, and will therefore be high in fibre.

Incomplete proteins There will be a lack of complete proteins due to the absence of meat in the diet.

A VEGAN DIET

A person on a vegan diet does not eat meat or dairy products, but uses milk, butter and cheese made from nuts and soya beans. Like vegetarians, vegans need to combine a range of plant foods in order to ensure that they are getting sufficient proteins. Due to the absence of certain foods from their diet, they may also need to take vitamin pill supplements (especially B12). If you are unsure whether or not vitamins are needed, consult a GP or nutritionist.

COMBINING PLANT FOODS

Unlike animal foods, no single plant food contains all the amino acids that the body requires. To assist their intake of 'complete' proteins, therefore, non-meat eaters need to make sure that they eat plant foods in the correct combinations.

Good combinations

Rice + Nuts or Seeds   Nuts or grains + Lentils

Beans or Peas + Cheese   Milk + Pasta

Bread + Beans or peas

CULTURAL DIETS

As a volunteer carer, you may be looking after someone whose beliefs are different from your own, so it is essential to understand their dietary needs. Fasting may be required on certain days, but in most cultures the infirm, elderly and babies are excluded from this, especially if the fast involves fluid deprivation. The actual dates for fasting may change from year to year.

SPECIAL CULTURAL REQUIREMENTS

CULTURE	DIETARY PREFERENCES	RESTRICTIONS
HINDU	• Many Hindus are vegetarian. • Beef is never eaten. • Cow's milk is acceptable. • Fasting is common, although fruit, salad without salt, and hot milk or tea are allowed.	• May object to utensils that have been used to prepare meat or meat products. • Some may abstain from alcohol & tobacco. **Special days in calendar:** Fasting on Ramanavami (1 day), Dushera (10 days) and Karva Chauth (1 day).
ISLAM	• Halal meat (from animals that have been ritually slaughtered according to Muslim law) is eaten. • Muslims do not eat pork or meat from other carnivorous animals.	• Halal meat should be stored and cooked separately from other products. • Some may abstain from alcohol & tobacco **Special days in calendar:** Fasting during Ramadan (30 days) from dawn to dusk, and Shab-E-Barat (1 day) three weeks before Ramadan begins.
JEWISH	• Kosher meat (blessed by a Rabbi and killed in a certain way) is preferred. • Orthodox Jews avoid pork, bacon, ham, rabbit and shellfish. • Meat and poultry must not be served with dairy products.	• Separate utensils must be used for dairy and meat products. • Three hours should elapse between eating meat and any dairy product. **Special days in calendar:** Fasting on Yom Kippur (25 hours) and food restrictions for Passover (8 days).
SIKHS	• Dairy produce is important. • Beef is never eaten. • Many Sikhs are vegetarian, but some can eat meat slaughtered following a rite called Chakardi.	• Some may abstain from alcohol & tobacco **Special days in calendar:** Some people, often women, fast; they do not avoid all foods, but may reduce the quantity or variety of food eaten for one to two days per week.
CHINESE	• Believe that health is related to a balance of the body's physical elements (Taoism).	• May think that cold food should not be eaten by an ill person or that an illness indicates a need to alter the diet.

MAKING MEALTIMES ENJOYABLE

Ideally, a balanced diet is made up of three meals a day but, if this is not possible, you should try to provide the equivalent amount of food and correct combination of nutrients on a daily basis. To encourage your relative to eat meals try to provide appetising food in a relaxed environment, and make sure she has the necessary items to enable her to eat without assistance.

PREPARING FOR A MEAL

To maximise enjoyment, make sure that your relative is comfortable and that she has everything she needs to hand. She should have enough room in which to eat her meal - whether she is sitting in a chair, or using a tray or bed table - and the food should look and taste as appetising as possible.

PROVIDE A RELAXED ENVIRONMENT

Listen to your relative's wishes: she may want music, or the television or radio turned on during her meal. Check whether she would like to use the toilet before eating, and offer her a chance to freshen up. You may want to consider freshening the room with flowers or potpourri. Eating in company can be more enjoyable than eating alone so, if it is convenient, you, or other members of the household, should join your relative for a meal.

ENSURE MEALS ARE APPETISING

Where possible, your relative should help to decide what is going to be cooked and, if she is able, be encouraged to help prepare the meal.

Think about what you give her Provide foods that she enjoys - and that she is allowed to eat - in small, manageable portions.

Make the food attractive Presentation is important with any meal and can encourage someone, who may otherwise have little appetite, to eat. Provide a choice of seasoning and pickles, but remember that some items such as salt, may not be permitted because of a medical condition. If it does not conflict with dietary restrictions, an alcoholic drink, such as a glass of sherry or wine before or with a meal, may stimulate her appetite.

PROVIDING FOOD FOR AN ILL PERSON

If your relative is ill, she may have little or no appetite. With short-term illnesses, such as a cold or mild flu, eating less is acceptable provided fluid intake is maintained. For long term illnesses, however, the right amount of food and the correct balance of nutrients is essential to help the body to fight disease and repair damage. If you are worried about the level of your relative's food intake, her GP or Public Health Nurse may suggest food supplements.

Quantity of food If your relative has lost her appetite, three large meals a day may prove daunting. It is better for her to eat a few small meals than to feel defeated because she cannot finish what is on her plate. Give her small, manageable portions throughout the day, and remove any leftovers immediately. Be patient and encouraging.

ADAPTING FOR A PHYSICAL IMPAIRMENT

Physical impairment does not necessarily mean that your relative cannot feed herself or enjoy her meals. You can encourage independence by obtaining special aids to suit her specific needs.

SOMEONE WITHOUT TEETH

If your relative is not able to wear dentures, she will find it difficult to chew, and will require a diet of soft foods. Prepare foods that can be mashed or use a mincer or liquidiser, if available.

SOMEONE WHO IS CONFINED TO BED

Make the person as comfortable as possible, using pillows to aid sitting. Place the items on a bed table or tray and check that the bedclothes are properly protected.

SOMEONE WHO CANNOT FEED HERSELF

If it is necessary to feed your relative, you can help to create a more relaxed atmosphere by talking and making her feel more comfortable. If you behave naturally, it will help to make both of you feel less self-conscious. When offering the food, make sure you hold the fork or spoon in your relative's line of vision so that she is able to see what she is eating.

CATERING HELP

If you are unable to provide meals, perhaps due to illness or because you are away from the house in the daytime, you may be able to get outside help. Seek advice from a care professional to find out what services are available in your area.

Meals on Wheels
This service provides a midday meal.

Day centres
If your relative attends a day centre, it is likely that she will be provided with a midday meal.

HELPING A VISUALLY IMPAIRED PERSON

Someone who is visually impaired should be able to feed herself, but thoughtful preparation will be required to enable her to be independent. Think about what you prepare - foods such as peas, for example, may be difficult for the person to eat as they slide around the plate.

The 'clock' method By simply arranging the food on the plate in a certain way, a visually impaired person can have more control over what she is choosing to eat. If she is told where the food is on the plate - for example, the potatoes are at '12 o' clock' - she will be able to eat without your assistance.

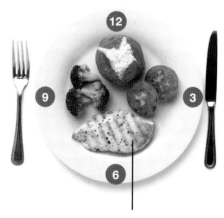

Place main item of food at '6 o'clock'

MINOR DIGESTIVE PROBLEMS

If your relative is ill she may vomit, especially after eating. Steps should be taken to limit any distress this may cause and, if the problem persists, medical help should be sought. An immobile person may have difficulty digesting food, which can lead to a variety of uncomfortable symptoms, collectively known as indigestion; as a result her diet and eating habits may need to be changed.

VOMITING

This may be a sign of an underlying illness or infection, so check for other symptoms. If vomiting occurs often, pass the following information to the GP:

- the colour and content of the vomit (check in particular for any blood);
- whether vomiting is linked to eating and drinking and;
- whether there is pain or diarrhoea.

To help, keep a bowl and flannel to hand and offer your relative the chance to freshen up afterwards.

EATING DISORDERS

Frequent vomiting can indicate eating disorders, such as anorexia nervosa or bulimia. Possible signs are:

- regular use of the lavatory after meals;
- avoiding meals altogether and;
- losing a lot of weight.

Seek medical advice if you suspect these disorders.

INDIGESTION AND HEARTBURN

Indigestion usually occurs soon after eating or drinking. The symptoms can vary, but there is often a feeling of fullness and discomfort in the abdomen, perhaps accompanied by belching, nausea and heartburn. Your relative should take preventive measures to avoid it occurring.

Pinpoint the cause Try to work out why the indigestion is occurring and avoid the cause, if possible.

Neutralise stomach acid Sometimes the discomfort is relieved by milk or an over-the-counter antacid (ask the pharmacist to recommend one), but the GP should be consulted if the symptoms persist or recur.

WHY INDIGESTION CAN OCCUR

If your relative's indigestion is due to her inability to chew, provide soft foods and seek the advice of her GP. Indigestion may also be caused by the following:

- lying down or bending forwards after eating a large meal;
- eating spicy meals;
- eating too quickly;
- drinking too much alcohol, or drinking alcohol on an empty stomach and;
- smoking.

Sites of discomfort

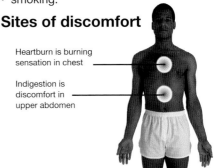

Heartburn is burning sensation in chest

Indigestion is discomfort in upper abdomen

CHAPTER 7

MAINTAINING & IMPROVING MOBILITY

Your relative's ability to walk or move about may be impeded as the result of an illness or injury, or simply because he is frail; either way he will be more reliant on you for help. There are varying degrees of immobility, ranging from difficulty in getting out of a chair to the inability to stand up or walk. An aid, such as a walking stick or walking frame, may enable your relative to undertake routine activities, such as shopping or visiting friends, by himself. This level of independence may greatly increase his confidence and assist in his recovery from illness.

TAKING CARE OF YOURSELF

There are strict guidelines for moving and handling an immobile person, which should be followed closely so that you avoid injuring yourself. If it is necessary for you to move your relative, ensure that the correct procedures are demonstrated to you by a healthcare professional, such as an occupational therapist, Public Health Nurse or physiotherapist. It is advisable that the carer undertakes a safe lifting course. If your relative is very immobile, there are special aids and equipment available that are designed to make it safer and easier for you to move him.

HANDLING SOMEONE SAFELY

If you attempt to move your relative incorrectly, you may injure yourself - particularly your back - or aggravate your relative's condition. These risks can be avoided if you follow the correct procedures for moving and handling a person. The techniques that are most appropriate for you and your relative should be demonstrated to you by a healthcare professional.

PREPARING TO MOVE SOMEONE

If part of your relative's daily care involves moving him, always make sure that you are fully prepared for the task. It is recommended in order to provide safe care for you and your patient that you take a course in safe lifting.

The move Is there anyone who can help you to move your relative?

You Have you been shown how to carry out the move? Are you wearing anything unsuitable - such as high-heeled shoes - which may be dangerous?

Your relative Is your relative mobile enough to help with part of the procedure; is he able to move himself to the edge of a chair, for example?

Safety Have you got enough space to carry out the procedure safely? Are you attempting any procedures that have not been fully explained to you?

HANDLING SOMEONE SAFELY

If you attempt to move someone incorrectly, you may injure yourself - particularly your back - or aggravate the person's condition.

- Do not move a person if you have a back injury;
- Do reassure the person and tell them what you plan to do;
- Do straighten your back when moving the person, and bend your knees, where necessary;
- Do wear supporting shoes with low heels;
- Only use equipment or moving and handling aids if their use has been fully demonstrated to you;
- Only move if absolutely necessary.

GETTING SPECIALIST HELP

If it is necessary to move your relative regularly, you must get specialist help. If you care for your relative on your own, it is especially important that you seek advice, as the risk of causing injury to yourself (particularly back strain), or to your relative, is increased.

Talking to a professional

The GP or Public Health Nurse can arrange for a specialist, such as a physiotherapist or an occupational therapist, to assess your situation and show you the correct procedures for moving and handling your relative.

Using equipment

If your relative needs a high level of assistance - if he has to be helped into a bed or a bath regularly, for example - you should be shown how to use specialist equipment, such as a hoist. You should also be shown how to maintain it.

WHEELCHAIRS

There are several different models of wheelchair available; the type recommended will depend on your relative's disability. Your local health professional will advise you.

When moving a wheelchair up or down a step or kerb, take your time so that the manoeuvre is safe. When tilting the chair, use the tipping lever.

GOING DOWN A STEP OR KERB

1 Face the step when approaching it. Tilt the wheelchair back by pushing down on the tipping lever with your foot.
2 With the chair tilted, push the back wheels to the edge of the kerb.
3 Push the chair down the kerb until the back wheels are on the ground. Then, lower the front wheels gently on to the ground.

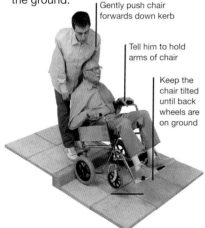

Gently push chair forwards down kerb

Tell him to hold arms of chair

Keep the chair tilted until back wheels are on ground

GOING UP A STEP OR KERB

1 Face the step when approaching it. Hold the handles securely. Place your foot on the tipping lever to tilt the chair backwards.
2 With the wheelchair balanced on its

rear wheels, push it forwards until the front wheels are resting on the pavement or on the upper level of the next step.
3 Use your body weight to push the wheelchair forwards and up the step until the back wheels are on the same level as the front. Never attempt to lift the wheelchair.

FOR A HEAVIER PERSON

There is a danger that a heavy occupant may fall out of the wheelchair if it is facing forwards when you push it down. You should, therefore, reverse the position and lower the chair backwards. For this manoeuvre, do not use the tipping lever to tilt the chair.

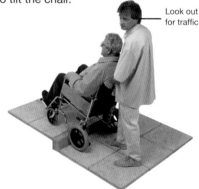

Look out for traffic

WHEELCHAIR SAFETY

To ensure your own safety and the safety of your relative, follow these guidelines:
• never attempt to lift the chair alone with someone in it;
• if the chair has a seat belt, make sure it is securely fastened when the chair is in use;
• do not push a wheelchair forwards down a step or kerb if the person in the chair is at all heavy;
• check brakes and tyre pressures regularly;
• make sure that the user is dressed safely and comfortably.

COMPLICATIONS OF IMMOBILITY

Prolonged immobility may adversely affect your relative's physical or mental health. As a carer, you need to be aware of the likely consequences, and know how to help prevent or alleviate them. As well as physical effects, debilitating conditions may lead to boredom, anger, depression and isolation, you will also need to provide emotional support and encourage recreational activities.

PHYSICAL EFFECTS OF IMMOBILITY

Immobility can sometimes lead to further complications, such as infections or poor circulation. It may be possible to minimise these complications by seeking the advice of the GP or Public Health Nurse and by following the suggestions below.

Urinary tract infections Sitting for long periods of time may prevent the bladder from emptying properly. Residual urine can stagnate in the bladder, which may result in infection. Encourage your relative to drink plenty of fluids to ensure urine flow.

Constipation Physical inactivity can lead to constipation, but a high-fibre diet and plenty of fluids can help to minimise this. If the problem persists, seek medical advice.

Chest infections Lying down for long periods causes mucus to stagnate in the lowest part of the chest. Regular changes of position and encouraging the person to take a number of deep breaths regularly can help to displace the mucus, so helping to prevent infection.

Circulatory problems Poor circulation can result from long periods of physical inactivity. Gentle physiotherapy may be recommended, or your relative may be prescribed special support stockings. If he complains of any sudden pains in his lower limbs or chest, tell the GP or Public Health Nurse immediately.

Pressure sores If your relative's condition results in him lying or sitting in one position for long periods, he is at risk of developing pressure sores. These occur in areas where skin and tissue are squeezed between the bones and an underlying surface; blood supply to the tissues is restricted so starving them of nutrients. To prevent pressure sores, an immobile person should change position at least every two hours. If pressure sores develop, seek urgent medical treatment. (See page 74)

ENCOURAGING MOBILITY

Even if a person has mobility problems, he should be encouraged to undertake some form of exercise to minimise the risk of any complications occurring. If your relative is confined to a wheelchair, seek advice from a healthcare professional about exercises designed specifically for wheelchair users.

Encouraging gentle exercise
Your relative should be encouraged to:
- undertake gentle exercise, such as short walks or swimming in a warm pool; these activities will help to improve his circulation;
- find out about local activities, such as sports or dancing, specifically arranged for people with disabilities;
- embark on or continue a hobby, such as gardening, that involves some form of exercise.

CHAPTER 8

BED COMFORT

Looking after someone who is confined to bed can be tiring and time-consuming for you, and frustrating and restrictive for the person affected.

MOVING A PERSON IN BED

You may have to help your relative into and out of bed, and even change her position once she is in bed. If you undertake these procedures incorrectly, you are in danger of injuring yourself and your relative. The effective ways of moving a person in bed should be demonstrated to you by a healthcare professional. If any specialist equipment is recommended, it is essential that you are shown how to use it correctly.

REST AND SLEEP

You can improve your relative's quality of life by making sure that she is as comfortable as possible in bed. There are also ways that you can minimise any physical discomfort or environmental disturbances that may prevent your relative getting essential rest and sleep.

BEDS AND BEDDING

Look at ways that your relative's existing bed can be adapted for her comfort and for your safety and convenience, as purchasing a new one may be disruptive for her. If your relative is in bed for long periods, you will need to change the bedding more often than usual. Make sure you have enough bed linen to be able to do this.

ADAPTING AND POSITIONING THE BED

To be able to care for someone effectively, the bed needs to be at the right height, not too wide and positioned so that you can reach both sides easily.

Bed height The mattress should be high enough for you to tend to your relative without having to bend too low. You may wish to use raisers to elevate the bed, but first seek professional advice.

Bed size It is easier to care for someone in a single bed so that you can reach her easily, without over stretching. If your relative prefers to sleep in a double bed, encourage her to lie on one side of it so that you can reach her more easily.

Position and location Position the bed away from the wall so that you can move around it easily. You may also need to relocate your relative's bedroom if she has difficulty climbing the stairs or so that she can get to the toilet more easily.

MAKING THE BED

When you need to change the sheets, encourage your relative to get out of bed. If she is not able to do this, use one of the methods shown opposite to make the bed. Whichever way you make the bed, bear in mind the following guidelines:

- remove all the bedding and replace it with clean linen, or transfer the top sheet to the bottom so that you only have to put on a clean top sheet;
- stretch the bottom sheet to the corners of the bed and smooth away any wrinkles; if left they could rub against the skin and cause pressure sores;
- tuck the top sheet in loosely to allow free movement of the feet, which can help to prevent pressure sores;
- keep a laundry basket close at hand for dirty linen.

SELECTING THE BEST BEDDING

Choose bed linen that is machine-washable easy to dry and comfortable.

Cotton covers Bed linen that is 100% cotton or a cotton mix is best, as it is less likely to cause a person to perspire. It can also be washed at high temperatures, whic is an important factor if the person has an infectious disease or is incontinent. You wil find fitted sheets easier to put on and keep flat.

Duvets Ideally, your relative should have two duvets: one with a low tog rating (the amount of thermal insulation it provides) fo the summer, and one with a heavier rating for the winter.

Incontinence bedding If you are caring for someone who is incontinent, it is advisable to obtain a mattress protector and/or a bec protector.

CHANGING SHEETS FOR A BEDRIDDEN PERSON

1 Roll up a clean sheet lengthways ready to use later. Turn the person on to his side. Roll the soiled sheet up to his back.

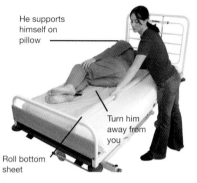

He supports himself on pillow

Turn him away from you

Roll bottom sheet

2 Place the rolled-up clean sheet on the edge of the bed, open end towards you. Unroll it to where the soiled sheet is placed.

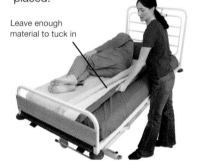

Leave enough material to tuck in

3 Turn the person towards you over the two rolls and on to the clean sheet. Remove the soiled sheet and place it in a washing bag or basket.

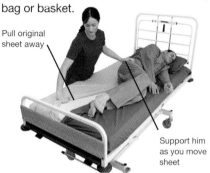

Pull original sheet away

Support him as you move sheet

4 Unroll the remainder of the clean sheet across the bed and tuck it in. Then turn him on to his back again and make him comfortable.

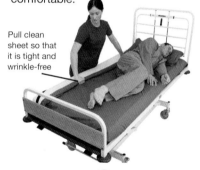

Pull clean sheet so that it is tight and wrinkle-free

FOR SOMEONE WHO CANNOT BE TURNED

If the person cannot lie on his side:
- sit him up;
- roll the dirty sheet up to his back;
- replace it with a clean sheet;
- move him back up the bed on to the clean sheet;
- remove the dirty sheet;
- pull the clean sheet from under his legs and tuck it in.

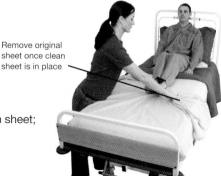

Remove original sheet once clean sheet is in place

AIDS TO COMFORT

In addition to suitable bedding, you may wish to seek advice from your Public Health Nurse or occupational therapist, who will be able to advise you on the choice of items that are most suitable for your relative's needs.

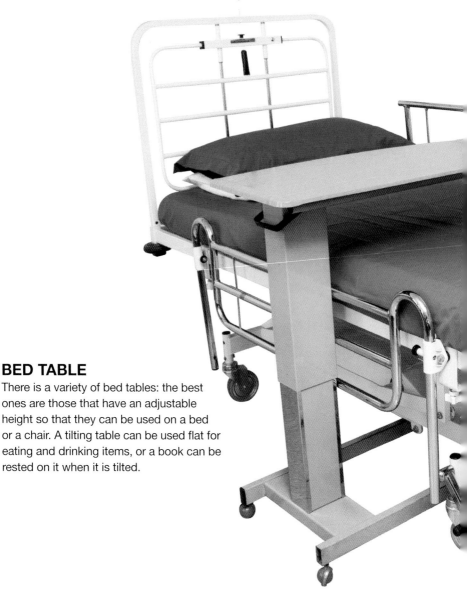

BED TABLE

There is a variety of bed tables: the best ones are those that have an adjustable height so that they can be used on a bed or a chair. A tilting table can be used flat for eating and drinking items, or a book can be rested on it when it is tilted.

MATTRESSES

Variable pressure relieving mattresses are available. These help distribute the person's weight evenly so that the points at which the body comes into contact with the mattress are varied, thus helping to prevent pressure sores.

V-SHAPED SUPPORT PILLOW

This is shaped to provide even support for the neck, back and arms.

Shaped to support arms

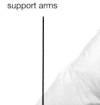

SUPPORTS

If your relative is confined to bed, it is essential that she sits up for some of the time. This is particularly important to prevent the onset of breathing difficulties and chest infections. To enable her to sit up, she must have adequate pillow support. Provide plenty of normal pillows, placing them under her head, neck, shoulders and arms for support, and consider purchasing one of the specialist varieties shown. For better support, the v-shaped pillow may need to be used in conjunction with ordinary pillows.

REST AND SLEEP

It is essential for your relative to get enough rest and sleep to restore energy, help the recovery process and improve morale. Get to know her sleep patterns and in times of wakefulness or restlessness, try to determine whether the cause is due to physical discomfort, anxiety or environmental disturbances. Sleeping pills should only be taken if prescribed by a doctor.

PHYSICAL AND PSYCHOLOGICAL DISCOMFORT

If your relative cannot get comfortable or relax, she may have difficulty sleeping. It is important that her bed is comfortable, that any pain or physical discomfort is minimised and that she is not kept awake by anxiety.

Make sure she has everything that she needs to hand, night-time medication and a drink, for example; this may help to minimise the length of time that she is kept awake. She may also like a book so that she can read herself to sleep.

SOLVING PHYSICAL AND EMOTIONAL PROBLEMS

PROBLEM	WHY IT OCCURS	SOLUTIONS
HUNGER OR THIRST	If a person wakes in the middle of the night, hunger and thirst can prevent her getting back to sleep.	Make sure she has enough to eat and drink during the day. Place a drink and snack on her bedside table at night.
PHYSICAL DISCOMFORT	The bed or bedding itself may be uncomfortable and aggravate physical problems. Wakefulness may also be caused by physical discomfort such as aching limbs, stiff joints or a full bladder.	Make your relative comfortable in bed. Check that bedding is not too heavy, sheets are not wrinkled or wet and pillows are a comfortable height. An immobile person should be provided with a toilet aid, such as a commode.
PAIN	Pain in the middle of the night may cause psychological as well as physical discomfort.	Make sure that she has taken the correct dosage of pain-relief medicine and that any painkillers required are to hand.
ANXIETY	A person may be kept awake because she is depressed or worried about her illness or a forthcoming operation.	Encourage your relative to talk about her concerns. Find ways for her to relax before bedtime, such as reading.

ENVIRONMENTAL DISTURBANCES

A change of environment may cause your relative to feel very disorientated, which can have a disruptive effect on sleep patterns. To minimise this, try to keep her bedtime routine as familiar as possible. If you have very noisy neighbours, explain to them that your relative needs to rest; you will find that most people will be sympathetic. It may also be worthwhile purchasing earplugs for your relative - they are available from chemists - especially if she likes to sleep during the day or goes to bed early.

SLEEP PATTERNS

Your relative should not become overtired, as this may hinder her recovery. Try to keep to her natural pattern of sleeping, and encourage her to follow this as closely as possible. If she is prevented from taking a customary nap in the afternoon, for example, she may want to sleep in the evening, which may then make it difficult for her to sleep during the night. Make sure that you are not deprived of sleep as well. If you get very tired, try to adapt your own sleep patterns around those of your relative: when she sleeps, use the opportunity to rest yourself.

MINIMISING ENVIRONMENTAL DISTURBANCES

PROBLEM	WHY IT OCCURS	SOLUTIONS
LIGHT	The room is too light or too dark at night.	If it is too dark, open the curtains or leave a light on. If it is too light, put up thicker curtains or line existing ones.
ODOURS	If the room has an intrusive smell it can disturb sleep.	Leave a window or door ajar so air can circulate.
CHANGE OF ENVIRONMENT	Your relative is not in her usual room, or has been relocated to a different building altogether.	If your relative is staying elsewhere, ensure that the rest of her bedtime routine remains as undisturbed as possible to minimise any disruption caused.
ROOM TEMPERATURE	Your relative is too hot or too cold at night.	Open or close windows and adjust heating and bedding as necessary; check her temperature.
NOISE	Noises outside and inside the house can disturb normal sleep patterns.	Try to remove the source of the noise; failing that, 'soundproof' the room by stuffing a rolled-up sheet or towel along the gap under the door.

PRESSURE SORES

When someone has to spend long periods of time in a bed or chair, she may be vulnerable to developing pressure sores. These sores occur in areas where the skin and underlying tissue are compressed between a surface and the bone, cutting off the blood supply to the affected area. Taking simple precautions can minimise the likelihood of pressure sores developing.

VULNERABLE AREAS

If your relative is weak or unconscious, and therefore unable to move in bed, there is a risk of pressure sores developing. These occur in places where the bones are very near the surface of the skin. The weight of the body reduces the blood supply to the skin tissues, causing the skin to change colour, initially to a pinky red. Areas that are vulnerable include:

- the head; • the shoulders;
- the elbows; • the base of the spine;
- the hips; • the heels and ankles.

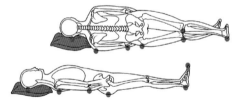

CAUSES OF PRESSURE SORES

Your relative may be vulnerable to pressures sores if:

- she remains in one position for too long;
- she has lost a lot of weight through illness, poor nutrition and therefore has less body fat to cushion the bones;
- there is friction on the skin, caused by the top sheet being too tight or by her being dragged across the bed, especially if her skin is not clean and dry.

WHAT ACTION YOU SHOULD TAKE

Pressure sores require swift medical attention. If you notice an area that is red, or one that appears blistered and tender, for over 24 hours, inform a healthcare professional, who will assess and determine what treatment is required. If the skin has broken, the sore is more prone to infection and may take longer to heal.

PREVENTING PRESSURE SORES

- encourage the person to get out of bed as much as possible;
- encourage her to move regularly. If she has very limited mobility, you will need to change her position every two hours;
- always move the person in the proper way; do not drag her limbs up or down the bed;
- never allow her to lie or sit in wet or damp conditions;
- make sure the bedding is not irritating the skin and wash the bedclothes regularly;
- following assessment by Public Health Nurse/Occupational Therapist/ Physiotherapist, specialist equipment may be advised;
- ensure that she is eating a balanced diet;
- inform the GP or Public Health Nurse about any skin changes, such as redness, dryness or cracking.

POSITIONS FOR BED REST

There are five basic positions for bed rest, all of which can be modified to suit individual needs. The patient's condition may dictate the best position for her, but her comfort is a prime consideration.

THE UPRIGHT POSITION (right)

The patient sits up with the back supported by several pillows, usually five, or by pillows and a backrest. Two of the pillows may be used to support her arms and a footrest used to prevent her from slipping down the bed.

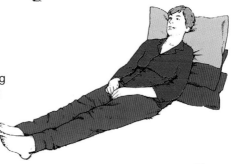

THE SEMI-RECUMBENT POSITION (right)

Three or four pillows support the patient's back. This is a comfortable position, allowing the patient to see around her and to eat and drink and converse without strain.

THE RECUMBENT POSITION (right)

The patient lies flat on her back with one or two pillows. This can be restful and allows her to turn on her side.

THE PRONE POSITION (right)

The patient lies face down with pillows to support her. This position is used for soreness of the back or buttocks.

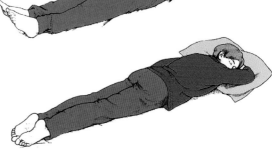

THE RECOVERY POSITION
(below)

This is used for the unconscious patient, who lies on his side with his lower leg stretched out behind and is prevented from rolling over by bending the upper leg and lower arms at right angles to the body. The patient's head rests on the hand of the upper arm as shown in the diagram. The head is turned to prevent the tongue blocking the airway. Note that there are no pillows - this is to prevent the patient inhaling his own vomit.

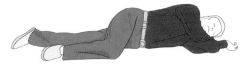

USING A DRAWSHEET

If the patient is in bed for more than a few days or is sweating a great deal, you may find a drawsheet useful. A drawsheet can be made from a rectangular piece of fabric about one metre wide and two metres long, or by folding a sheet in half lengthways. It is then placed on top of the bottom sheet under the patient's buttocks, and allows a clean cool area to be moved under the patient without there being any need to change the bottom sheet.

When you are making the bed, place the drawsheet on top of the bottom sheet. Tuck in one side, pull the sheet taut at the other side and tuck in the end first, then the slack. When the patient is uncomfortable and you want to adjust the drawsheet, untuck it at both ends. Pull a fresh area under the patient's buttocks, then tuck in at both sides again. The length of the drawsheet allows three or four clean areas to be pulled through before the sheet needs changing.

CHANGING A DRAWSHEET

1 Roll a clean drawsheet up from one short edge. Roll the patient on to their side and have someone to help support them. Roll up the soiled drawsheet. Tuck in the clean drawsheet and unroll it until it meets the soiled one. Roll the patient over both sheets, remove the soiled one and gather the clean one in loose folds on the bed.

2 Tuck in the end, pull out the folds and allow the slack to drop down. Pull taut and tuck in.

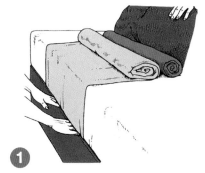

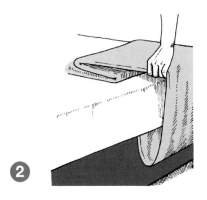

CHAPTER 9

PERSONAL CARE

It is essential to your relative's self-esteem and self-respect that he is able to maintain a good standard of personal hygiene and dress himself. This will help to make him feel better about himself and to cope more positively with his condition.

ENCOURAGING INDEPENDENCE

Your support and encouragement are essential, especially if he is relearning basic skills that he once took for granted, such as brushing his teeth or putting on socks and shoes. Encourage him to carry out as many of the tasks as he can on his own and resist the urge to help, even if he is taking a long time.

HELPING YOUR RELATIVE

It may be necessary for you to help your relative to wash and dress. In this situation you need to find the safest and easiest ways to do this and, if necessary, seek advice from a healthcare professional, such as a Public Health Nurse or an occupational therapist. If your relative is confined to bed, you may be shown how to give a bed bath; if he has severe mobility problems and you do not have a shower cubicle, an occupational therapist may recommend the use of equipment to help you to move him into and out of the bath.

HELPING SOMEONE TO WASH

Always encourage your relative to, at the very least, wash his hands and face at a basin by himself. If he has mobility problems or is weak, you may have to adapt the bathroom to enable him to use it by himself. If it is necessary to help him into a bath, always seek advice about the safest way to do this; an adapted shower cubicle may be a safer option.

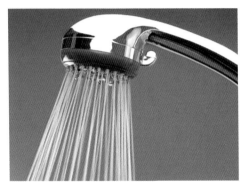

HELPING SOMEONE TO HAVE A SHOWER

An immobile person who cannot climb into a bath should be encouraged to use a shower cubicle. If he has difficulty standing in the shower, obtain a shower seat; if he is confined to a wheelchair, a chair can be obtained that can be wheeled into and out of the cubicle. It is also advisable to fit handrails and get a non-slip mat for the floor.

You can help your relative by:
• ensuring that he has all his toiletries;
• turning on the water and making sure it is the correct temperature;
• passing the shower head once he is securely seated. Leave him alone, unless he needs assistance and supervision throughout. Agree, beforehand, on a way to communicate that he has finished.

HELPING SOMEONE TO HAVE A BATH

If your relative cannot climb into the bath by himself, you may have to help him. You must not, however, attempt to lift him into or out of the bath. Seek the advice of a healthcare professional, who may suggest the use of specialist equipment, such as a hoist or bath lift, to enable you to move him. If your relative's mobility is only slightly impaired - just generally weak, for example - he may benefit from the use of some simple aids.

Grab rails The person can hold on to these as he gets into and out of the bath.

Non-slip mat This is placed in the bottom of the bath to prevent the person slipping while getting in and out and while sitting in the bath.

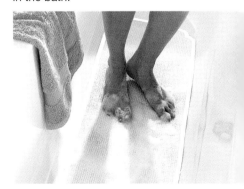

GIVING SOMEONE A BED BATH

Your relative will require a bed bath if he is unable to get out of bed to wash. You will need a bowl of warm water, two or three towels, soap and two sponges or flannels; use different sponges for the face and genitals. Keep him warm by covering those parts of the body that are not being washed with a sheet and towel.

1 Remove the person's upper-body clothing. Pull the top sheet up to his armpits and cover it with a towel. Wash his face, neck, shoulders, arms and hands, and then dry these areas.

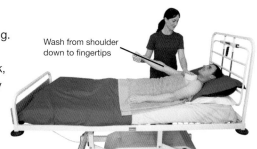

Wash from shoulder down to fingertips

2 Fold the sheet and towel down to his waist. Wash and dry his chest and abdomen; make sure that you dry thoroughly under any folds of skin as sores may develop in areas that remain damp or wet.

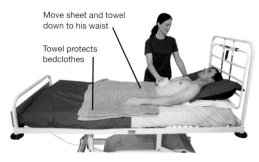

Move sheet and towel down to his waist

Towel protects bedclothes

3 Cover the top half of his body. Remove any lower-body clothing. Wash and dry his legs and feet. Allow him to wash the genital area himself with the second sponge. Cover him with the sheet, while you change the water.

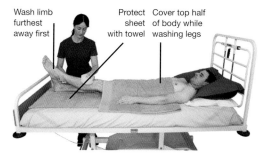

Wash limb furthest away first

Protect sheet with towel

Cover top half of body while washing legs

4 Turn the person on to his side. Use the original sponge to wash his back and buttocks. Dry him and help him dress into clean clothes. If someone has difficulty lying on his side, sit him up. Protect the bottom sheet with a towel and then wash and dry his back.

CARE OF GENERAL APPEARANCE

As well as staying clean, it may be important to your relative's self-esteem to look as presentable as possible - even if he is feeling unwell. If your relative is female, applying make-up does not have to be part of her daily routine if she does not want it to be, but when people are visiting, or when she is going out shopping or to the day centre, it may help to boost her confidence.

APPLYING MAKE-UP

You can obtain several useful items that can help your relative to apply make-up without your help.

Magnifying mirror A closer and clearer view can be achieved with a magnifying mirror propped up on a stand for easy use.

Foam tubing Specialist tubing can be attached to items such as lipsticks, eye pencils and mascaras, to make them easier to grip and thereby easier to apply.

Make-up bag Attach a long ring pull to the zip on a make-up bag, or replace the zip with velcro, so that someone who has difficulty gripping can open and close it easily.

Containers It may be better to purchase creams and lotions in pots, as a person with limited dexterity may find it difficult to squeeze a tube.

HELPING SOMEONE TO SHAVE

If you are caring for a man, you may need to help him shave. Always ask him whether he would prefer a wet shave or an electric shave. An electric razor may be easier for you to use if you are not practised or confident in the art of giving a wet shave. Always ensure that the equipment is clean.

GIVING A WET SHAVE

You will need a razor, shaving cream or soap and water. Rub the soap or foam into a lather over the area to be shaved. The person may be able to do this himself. Then, hold the skin taut with one hand and firmly pull the razor down the cheek in long strokes. The razor should be sharp enough to cut the stubble and not scrub across his face. Rinse the razor after every few strokes. Rinse the face when you have finished.

USING AN ELECTRIC RAZOR

The hand-over-hand method gives some independence to a person who is able to grip an electric razor, but unable to rotate it. Once he is holding the razor, place your hand over his to direct it.

Using the hand-over -hand method

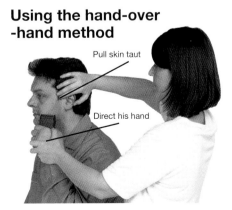

Pull skin taut

Direct his hand

CARING FOR THE HAIR

Clean and groomed hair, even if it is just simply brushed to remove tangles and styled so that it is neat and manageable, may have a significant effect on how your relative feels about himself. A hairwash, especially, can be very refreshing and uplifting. Regular haircuts will make hair easier to manage - if your relative is housebound, find a hairdresser who can come to your home.

GENERAL HAIR CARE

Unless your relative is very weak, they should be encouraged to brush or comb their hair by themselves.

Brushing hair If your relative's condition means that they have to lie or sit in the same position for long periods of time, their hair may become tangled. Lying on tangled hair may cause the scalp to become sore, possibly resulting in pressure sores. To prevent this occurring, encourage your relative to brush or comb their hair gently, at least twice a day.

Wig care Your relative may have had treatment that has led to hair loss, such as chemotherapy. If they wish to wear a wig, consult a specialist for advice. Wash artificial wigs by hand; natural hair wigs should be washed and styled by a hairdresser.

WASHING THE HAIR

Having the hair washed can be very refreshing for someone who is ill. Your relative should wash their hair in the bath or shower, if possible. Ask the pharmacist for a dry shampoo or no-rinse shampoo so that they can keep their hair clean between washes.

For someone confined to bed

If your relative cannot get up, you can obtain a device to wash their hair while lying in bed.

Alternatively, you can wash it by:
- laying plastic sheeting or towels over the bed and floor;
- positioning the person so that they are sitting up and leaning over a bowl on a bed table. If it is difficult for them to sit up, they can lie with their head over the bottom end of the bed, pillows under their neck and shoulders, and a bowl beneath their head.

HAIRWASHING TRAY

This inflatable tray allows a person to lie flat while his hair is being washed; it is especially useful for someone who has very limited mobility. Place a bowl beneath the hose to collect the water that drains from the tray.

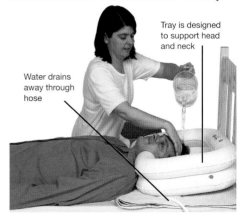

Tray is designed to support head and neck

Water drains away through hose

GENERAL BODY CARE

Medication, some courses of treatment and general immobility may lead to uncomfortable physical side effects. Many of the more common complaints, such as mouth ulcers and eye infections, are treatable at home, as the chart below indicates. There may also be steps you can take to prevent the side effects occurring in the first place. Always seek medical advice, if necessary.

TREATING AND PREVENTING COMMON COMPLAINTS

AREA	COMMON COMPLAINTS	RECOMENDED CARE
MOUTH	• Cheek and gum ulcers caused by poor-fitting dentures. • Lack of or excessive salivation, possibly as the result of a stroke. • Poor oral hygiene, cold sores, dehydration and dry tongue.	• Consult a dentist about getting new dentures for your relative. • Provide plenty of fluids and fresh fruit to encourage salivation. • Encourage your relative to brush her teeth thoroughly and provide mouth washes.
EYES	• Difficulty blinking or closing the eyes as a result of a stroke. • Eye infection and dry eyes.	• Wash around the eyes carefully from nose outwards, use new swab for each eye. • Drops or ointments may be prescribed to treat infection.
NOSE	• Blocked nose and sore nostrils from cold symptoms.	• Drops may be prescribed to relieve congestion, or creams to soothe soreness.
FEET	• Corns, bunions and blisters. • Fungal infections, such as athlete's foot. • Pressure sores.	• Seek the advice of the GP for fungal infections, otherwise consult a chiropodist. • Take steps to prevent pressure sores and seek medical advice.
NAILS	• Hard, brittle nails, prone to splitting, on fingers and toes. • Ingrowing toenails.	• Seek the advice of a chiropodist. • Trim nails regularly, cutting straight across and not down into the corners.
EARS	• Excessive wax, which may be soft or hard. • Sores on the edge of the ears.	• Drops may be prescribed. • Take steps to prevent pressure sores and seek medical advice.
SKIN	• Red, sore skin in the armpits, groin or breast areas. • Dry, flaky skin. • Rash caused by allergy	• Ensure skin in these areas is kept dry. • Moisturise regularly. • Seek medical advice - an emollient cream may be prescribed.

HELPING SOMEONE TO DRESS

Dressing and undressing can be a lengthy process for a weak or paralysed person. If possible, allow your relative to dress independently, but if he needs help, follow these guidelines:

- make sure he is sitting or lying down to make the task easier;
- dress the weak limb first;
- always place a garment over the arm before pulling it over the head;
- allow him to assist, if at all possible, but do not rush him.

HELPING TO PUT ON SOCKS

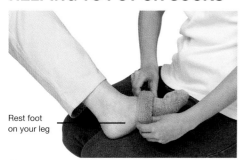

Rest foot on your leg

1 Fold over the top of the sock. Roll it back to halfway along the foot section and place it over the toes.

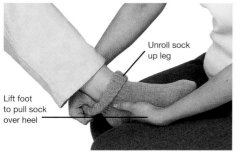

Unroll sock up leg

Lift foot to pull sock over heel

1 Supporting the underneath of the foot, unroll the sock over the foot, heel and up the leg.

DRESSING A PERSON WHO HAS AN INJURED ARM

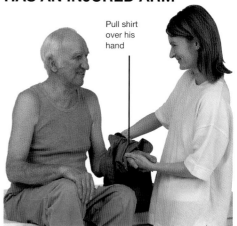

Pull shirt over his hand

1 Roll the sleeve down to the cuff. Place your hand through the cuff opening and take hold of the person's hand. Pull the shirt from your own hand over his.

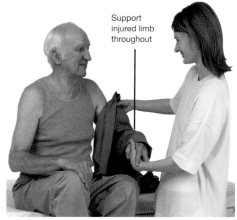

Support injured limb throughout

2 Keep hold of his hand and gently pull the shirt sleeve up his arm to the shoulder.

3 Take the garment around his back, so that he can reach the other sleeve with his good arm. He can then continue dressing by himself.

CHOOSING CLOTHES

Ideally, let your relative choose the clothes he would like to wear; if he relies on you to buy them, always opt for colours and fabrics that you know he likes. As well as buying items that are comfortable, consider what is practical: for example, if your relative has dexterity problems, do not buy garments with small buttons or back pockets.

FEATURES TO LOOK FOR

Choose items that may enable a person to dress without help. For example:
- slip-on shoes;
- v-necked jumper;
- sweatshirt or T-shirt;
- wrapover and skirt;
- clip-on tie.

If your relative has dexterity problems or is weak, consider how easy he will find it to manipulate the fastenings on garments.

FOR WHEELCHAIR USERS

People who use a wheelchair often find that their waist and hips broaden; users of manual chairs find that their shoulder and upper arm muscles also get bigger. It may, therefore, be necessary for them to wear larger clothing. For safety and comfort, the following are advised:

- close-fitting sleeves and cuffs to avoid catching fabric in the wheels;
- longer-length skirts for a woman so that they fall easily over her knees when she is seated;
- short coats or jackets so that the person is not sitting on them; long coats can also get caught in the wheels;
- low-heeled, well-fitting shoes with non-slip soles, as these are less likely to slip off the footrests;
- short scarves that can be tied easily so that they don't get caught in the wheels.

SIMPLE FASTENINGS

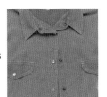

Press studs Press studs (poppers) are fastened by pressing together both halves. Use instead of buttons.

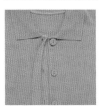

Large buttons Small buttons can be fiddly and difficult to grip. Choose garments with large buttons or replace small ones and widen the buttonholes.

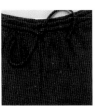

Drawstring waist Choose garments that have an elasticated waist. A drawstring is easy to tie and untie and an elasticated waist is more comfortable.

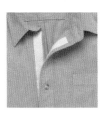

Velcro This consists of two nylon surfaces that stick to each other when pressed together. Replace buttons with velcro and resew them over the buttonholes.

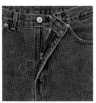

Invisible zip pull The catch is attached through the hole in the zip tag. The zip is moved by pulling the loop, which can then be tucked away.

CHAPTER 10

BLADDER & BOWEL CONTROL

Problems that affect the bladder and bowel are very common and range from constipation, diarrhoea, incontinence and abnormalities of the urinary and lower digestive tract.

INCONTINENCE

Looking after a person who has either poor control or lost control of their bladder or bowel - a condition known as incontinence - is possibly one of the most difficult tasks for any carer. Incontinence occurs when illness, injury or degeneration disturbs normal bladder or bowel function, leading to the involuntary discharge of urine or faeces. Incontinence is an indication that something has gone wrong with the normal functions of the bladder or bowel. Those affected and their carers often feel distressed and embarrassed by their situation, are often unwilling to discuss their problem with anyone, and so may become isolated and left to cope on their own.

TREATMENTS

Most bladder and bowel problems can be treated successfully or can be significantly improved so medical advice should always be sought. Solutions range from pelvic floor exercise programmes, to dietary and environmental changes, medication and possible surgical intervention. Before any treatment programme is commenced it is important that a General Practitioner, Continence Adviser or a Public Health Nurse carries out an assessment.

MINOR CONDITIONS

Bladder and bowel conditions, which include urinary problems, constipation and diarrhoea, may be the symptom of an underlying illness, an infection or a treatment. If your relative complains of any change in her bladder or bowel movements, such as frequency, discomfort or discolouration, or she has any difficulty in going to the toilet, you should always seek advice from a GP, Public Health Nurse or Continence Adviser.

RECOGNITION AND TREATMENTS

Once you recognise that there is a problem, you can identify possible causes and explore treatments.

WHAT TO DO FOR URINARY PROBLEMS

Your relative may have an infection if passing urine causes stinging and discomfort, or if the urine:
- is dark or cloudy in colour, or contains blood;
- has a particularly pungent smell;
- is being passed in small quantities frequently.

Seek medical help Your relative's GP may need to prescribe medication to treat the infection if it is the cause of the urinary problem.

WHAT TO DO FOR CONSTIPATION

This condition occurs when the person has failed to open her bowels as normal. There may be an obstruction, or the waste matter (faeces) may have become dry, making it difficult to pass.

Seek medical help A doctor may prescribe laxatives, suppositories or, in severe cases, an enema.

Encourage toilet use Encourage your relative to use the toilet regularly, even though she may be reluctant to do so because her bowel movements are painful.

Adapt the diet Make sure she eats a balanced diet and drinks plenty of fluids, especially water.

WHAT TO DO FOR DIARRHOEA

When a person passes liquid faeces at frequent intervals, the condition is known as diarrhoea.

Seek medical help The advice of a GP should be sought, especially if the person is elderly or ill.

Adapt the diet Give your relative plenty of fluids, including water. Abstaining from food for 24 hours may also help to relieve diarrhoea.

URINATION & DEFECATION

Someone who is healthy will pass urine and faeces naturally. How urine is passed:
- the bladder stores urine produced in the kidneys;
- as the bladder fills, nerve impulses signal to the brain that the bladder is full and must be emptied;
- the urine is passed - and discharged - through a tube (the urethra) connected to the bladder

How faeces are passed:
- digestion takes place as food passes from the stomach to the small intestine;
- any nutrients are absorbed into the bloodstream; what remains passes into the large bowel;
- this waste matter (faeces), which is no longer required by the body, is stored in the large bowel before being expelled via the rectum.

INCONTINENCE

Incontinence is surprisingly common amoung men and women of all ages and is not just a disease of the older adult. Four in ten women and one in ten men will suffer from incontinence at some stage during their life. If your relative is incontinent consult a General Practitioner, Continence Adviser or a Public Health Nurse to find an effective way to manage and treat the problem.

CAUSES AND TREATMENTS

CAUSE	WHAT HAPPENS	TREATMENT
INFECTION	• Someone who has an infection may have a strong urge to urinate followed by an involuntary emptying of the bladder. Passing urine may be painful, causing a burning sensation.	• Medication to treat the infection. • Sufficient fluid intake.
CONSTIPATION	• Faeces become impacted in the rectum; liquid faeces may seep out. In some cases, the resulting pressure on the bladder may lead to urinary incontinence.	• A high fibre diet with fresh fruit and vegetables. • Drink a minimum of 6-8 cups of fluids per day and cut down on tea/coffee /fizzy drinks. • Do not use laxatives long term unless directed by GP. • Correct toilet positioning stimulates motion.(See diagram page 93). • If problem persists consult GP.
ENLARGED PROSTATE	• The enlarged prostate gland blocks the passage of urine. The bladder fills up and then involuntarily releases an overflow of urine.	• Insertion of a catheter. • Medication. • Surgery or other treatment to remove or resect the prostate gland.

CAUSES AND TREATMENTS (CONT...)

CAUSE	WHAT HAPPENS	TREATMENT
WEAK MUSCLE TONE/ STRESS INCONTINENCE	• The muscles that control the passing of urine or faeces become weak so that urine (and, rarely, faeces) is passed involuntarily after coughing, sneezing or mild exercise. In women it is associated with pregnancy, childbirth, constipation and menopause. In men it is generally due to problems with the prostrate gland.	• Pelvic floor exercise. • Toilet routine. • Medication. • Surgery.
OVERACTIVE BLADDER	• 'Urgency' occurs when a person has a sudden strong urge to pass urine. They may also need to go very often (more than 8 times a day) or they may wet the bed. This can be caused by an overactive bladder muscle, infection, medication, poor mobility, constipation and in men enlarged prostate gland.	• Limit the intake of tea, coffee, alcohol and sugary drinks as these can irritate the bladder. • Pelvic floor exercises. • Bladder retraining. • Medication.
DAMAGE TO NERVOUS SYSTEM	• If the nervous system is damaged, for example paralysis, the person may be unable to recognise his need to use the toilet.	• Encourage toilet use, make sure that your relative goes, or is taken every 2 - 3 hours. • Use reminders, i.e. set an alarm clock. • Bladder retraining. • Insertion of a catheter. • Intermittent self-catherisation.
DEMENTIA	• A person may have normal bladder and bowel function, but be unable to get to the toilet in time, or need help once there. With dementia she may also be unable to express the need to go. Changes in the environment may disorientate.	• Toilet routine and reminders. • Use of toilet aids with supervision. • Sign posting on doors.

CAUSES AND TREATMENTS (CONT...)

CAUSE	WHAT HAPPENS	TREATMENT
PHYSICALLY IMPAIRED	• Bladder and bowel function may be normal but the person may be unable to get to the toilet on time, or have difficulty in removing their clothes.	• Provide practical clothes. • Ensure that an immobile person's living and sleeping quarters are near to the toilet. • Use toilet aids.
BED WETTING (ENURESIS)	• This is a common problem that can affect 10% of 5 year olds, 5% of 10 year olds and 1 - 2% of adults. Bed wetting occurs when the bladder is full but the 'wake up and hold on' signal does not get through to the brain.	• Talk to your GP or specialist nurse who will refer you to the Enuresis Clinic. • Drink plenty of fluids throughout the day, before the evening. • Bladder retraining. • Enuresis alarms. • Medication.
OVERFLOW	• In some people the bladder may not empty completely. Urine builds up and may lead to overflow. The most common causes are obstruction of the urine pathway, enlarged prostate gland, constipation and nerve damage (See page 91).	• Bladder retraining. • Surgery or other treatment.

PROMOTING CONTINENCE

Most incontinence can be treated and many people can be completely cured or show considerable improvement. The assessment by a GP, Continence Adviser or Public Health Nurse will pinpoint why the incontinence occurs and the correct treatment plan can be put in place to alleviate or contain the problem. In certain circumstances incontinence wear may be recommended following assessment of bladder and bowel problems.

WHAT CAN BE DONE TO HELP?

Before any treatment programme is commenced it is important that an assessment is carried out.

PELVIC FLOOR EXERCISES

Pelvic floor exercises will strengthen the weakened muscle and improve bladder control. Everybody is different and needs an exercise programme to suit their individual needs. It is important to get instructions from a Physiotherapist, Continence Adviser or Public Health Nurse.

BLADDER RETRAINING

Bladder retraining will help people with urgency/urge incontinence. The bladder may have become used to holding small amounts of urine and the signal to empty will happen more frequently. It might be helpful not to respond to the first signal to urinate, but to practice holding on, thus increasing the time span between toileting. After 3-4 weeks the urgency should reduce.

MEDICATION

Medication can help sometimes but can also cause urgency/urge incontinence.

Most often medication is used to:
- Reduce urge incontinence;
- Treat bladder infections;
- Stimulate the kidneys to pass urine e.g. fluid tablets (diuretics) and;
- Medication can also cause constipation.

COPING EMOTIONALLY

Incontinence can be a very difficult problem to cope with and, sadly, it is one of the main reasons why people give up their caring role. The problem is aggravated when the person does not admit to the problem and tries to cover up accidents by hiding soiled clothes, or when she appears to be incontinent on purpose. Before you can begin to deal with the problem, whatever its cause, it is important for both of you to be honest about how you feel.

Your feelings It is very normal to feel angry and disgusted by having to deal with incontinence. If you are finding it difficult to cope, seek help. Trying to cope alone will not be beneficial for either you or your relative.

Your relative's feelings It is very likely to be embarrassing and frustrating for your relative if she has to rely on you because she is unable to carry out these most basic of functions. Allow her as much privacy and independence as possible. Encourage her to talk about it and try to be understanding.

HELPFUL HINTS FOR PROMOTING CONTINENCE

It is normal to go to the toilet 7 times a day and maybe 1-2 times per night for an older adult. The hints below are designed to help you give guidance on how to help your relative to be continent.

- Restricting fluid intake does not help. In fact it can make the incontinence worse.
- Tea, coffee and fizzy drinks stimulate the bladder and should be reduced or avoided.
- The toilet should be readily accessible.
- A commode or urine bottle beside the bed at night might also be useful.
- Specialist equipment for the toilet and advice on its suitability can be obtained from the Public Health Nurse or Occupational Therapist.
- In certain circumstances incontinence wear may be recommended following assessment of bladder and bowel problems.
- Good personal hygiene reduces the risk of skin problems and unpleasant odours.
- Don't be afraid to seek medical advice.
- Correct toilet positioning stimulates motion and is important to prevent constipation (see diagram).

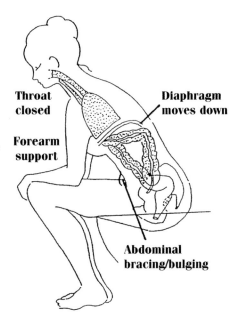

Throat closed

Diaphragm moves down

Forearm support

Abdominal bracing/bulging

INCONTINENCE AIDS

There is a range of aids to help with incontinence. Ask to see a continence adviser, who will be able to assess the extent of your relative's problem, taking her age and mental and physical condition into account. He or she will also be able to give you advice on the devices most likely to help your relative, and provide information on diet and available supports.

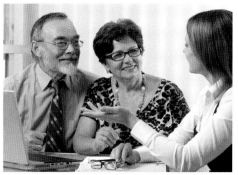

ALARM CLOCK

An alarm clock is useful if your relative does not recognise his need to go to the toilet. To establish a routine, set the alarm to go off every 2–3 hours as a reminder that it is time to use the toilet.

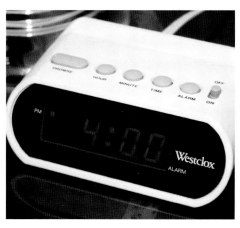

PADS

Incontinence pads There are designs for men and women, and a variety of sizes and absorbency levels. They can be used with or without special pants. The pad, which works on the same principle as a nappy, will absorb moisture and ensure that the wearer's skin remains dry.

ADAPTING AN INCONTINENT PERSON'S DIET

In some cases, adapting your relative's diet and fluid intake can help to control incontinence.

Food A high-fibre diet can help to prevent constipation, which may be the cause of faecal incontinence.

Fluid Limiting drinks in the evening may help if the urinary incontinence tends to occur at night. Do not, however, try to deal with urinary incontinence by limiting fluid intake during the day. It is essential to your relative's health that she drinks sufficient fluids.

BEDDING FOR AN INCONTINENT PERSON

There is a wide variety of incontinence products available, from mattress and pillow protectors to incontinence sheets. There are different types of absorbency to suit the level of incontinence. You may not need all the items shown below; a continence adviser will recommend those most suitable for your relative. Where possible, choose bedding that is easy to wash and dry. A mattress protector may cause some people to sweat excessively; discontinue use if this happens. For your relative's comfort, and to prevent sores developing, always change wet bedding as quickly as possible. If you are using specialist absorbing protection change according to manufacturers guidelines.

PROTECTING BEDDING

1 Place a fitted waterproof protector over the mattress.

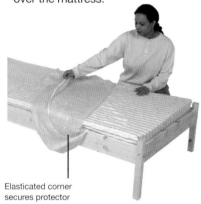

Elasticated corner secures protector

2 Put an ordinary bottom sheet on top of the protector and tuck it in securely.

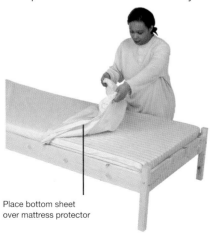

Place bottom sheet over mattress protector

3 Strip the pillow of its cover and replace it with a waterproof protector. Put an ordinary pillowcase over the protector.

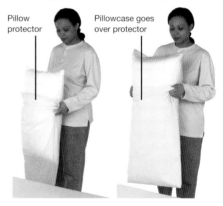

Pillow protector

Pillowcase goes over protector

4 Place an absorbent bed protector over the bottom sheet.

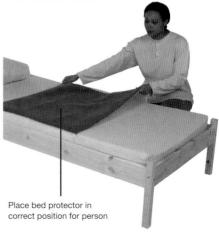

Place bed protector in correct position for person

TOILET AIDS

If your relative is immobile or confined to bed, she may benefit from the use of a toilet aid, such as a urinal, commode or bed pan. These aids will help to reduce the risk of having an 'accident', and give a degree of independence when using the toilet.

USING SPECIAL TOILETS

When your relative wants to use a urinal, commode or bed pan, make sure:
- she is able to unbutton or remove the necessary clothing easily;
- there is a toilet roll to hand;
- she can be left in private, if possible.

After using the toilet, establish a way for your relative to communicate to you that she has finished, then:
- assist her to clean herself, if she is unable to do this on her own;
- ensure that she washes her hands;
- wash the equipment;
- wash your hands.

Urinals These are mainly used by men, but the pan type can be used by women, and is good for wheelchair use.
How to help Encourage your relative to use it alone, but if she is unable to do so, help her. It is difficult for a man to use a urinal lying down, so he may need to sit supported on the edge of the bed.

MALE URINAL

Flip-top prevents leakages after use

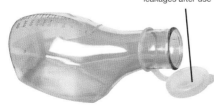

Commode

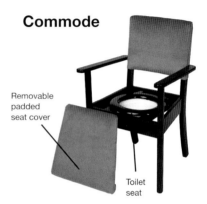

Removable padded seat cover

Toilet seat

Commodes These are chairs with a removable seat that conceals a built-in commode pan and toilet seat. Easy to clean, commodes are ideal for those who can get out of bed, but cannot get to the toilet.
How to help Help the person on to the commode, and give her as much privacy as her condition allows.

Bed pans These are used for a person who cannot get out of bed. The wedge-shaped slipper type is particularly easy to use, allowing the person to slide backwards and lift herself on to it.
How to help If it is a steel pan, make sure it is warm and dry. Ask her to raise herself, or help her to do this, then slide the bed pan underneath her. Provide a man with a urinal as well.

Slipper bed pan

Wedge-shaped for easier positioning

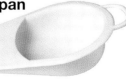

MEDICAL TREATMENTS

It may be necessary for a person with bladder and bowel problems to be fitted with a device that allows urine or faeces to be passed and collected through a different channel: a catheter for someone with urinary incontinence, or a stoma with a bag for someone with a disease of the digestive tract. If properly maintained, these can enhance the person's quality of life.

CATHETER CARE

As part of the medical treatment for a bladder problem or as a last resort for untreatable incontinence, a tube (catheter) may be inserted into the bladder to drain urine. The tube is then attached to a collecting bag strapped to the person's leg.

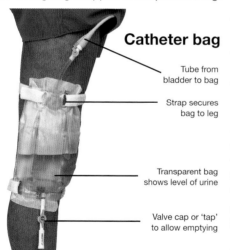

Catheter bag

Tube from bladder to bag

Strap secures bag to leg

Transparent bag shows level of urine

Valve cap or 'tap' to allow emptying

LOOKING AFTER THE CATHETER

Most catheters are inserted into the bladder and left in place. The person will be shown when and how to empty the bag. The tube is replaced at varying intervals by a GP or Public Health Nurse. People with intermittent incontinence, such as those with multiple sclerosis, may be taught how to do intermittent self-catherisation. To prevent infection, the person should wash the area around the catheter every day with soap and water, and drink plenty of fluids. You should understand the washing and emptying procedures, as you may have to assist your relative.

EMPTYING A CATHETER BAG

The bag should be emptied approximately every four hours or if it is more than two-thirds full.

Draining the bag The cap at the bottom of the bag is opened and the urine is drained into a container kept for this purpose. The urine is flushed down the toilet. If the bag is supplied separately, it may have to be changed. Follow instructions carefully and wear gloves to minimise the risk of infection. **Checking the tube** After emptying, the tube that leads from the catheter to the bag should be checked to make sure it is not kinked or blocked.

DEALING WITH COMPLICATIONS

A catheter may cause a urinary infection. If your relative complains of a burning sensation when urinating and/or has cloudy urine, it may indicate an infection. Always seek medical help. If the catheter actually comes out, no attempt should be made to reinsert it as this may seriously damage the bladder or urethra. If complications arise, seek advice from a Continence Adviser, Public Health Nurse or GP.

STOMA CARE

When the digestive tract is diseased or damaged in some way, or it is not possible for the person to pass faeces normally, surgery may be necessary.

The stoma Part of the large intestine (a colostomy) or small intestine (an ileostomy) can be brought out on to the abdomen to form an opening (stoma). The size of the stoma may vary in size and colour. It will be quite red and swollen, but may become smaller and turn pink. A specialist bag is fitted over the stoma to collect faeces. It may still be possible for a person who has a temporary stoma to pass faeces in the normal way.

SPECIALIST ADVICE

Before and after the operation, the person will be cared for by a stoma care nurse. The best position for the stoma will be discussed, although it may not always be possible to decide on the site beforehand. The nurse will also provide information about the operation and advice on aftercare.

AFTERCARE

A stoma should not prevent a person from leading a normal life. Stoma bags are very well designed and are not noticeable even under shorts or a swimsuit. If the correct aftercare is given, normal bowel movement should return, enabling the person to resume a full and active life. The person will need to follow specialist advice on changing the bag, skin care and diet. As the carer, you can help by making sure that there is an adequate supply of bags - these are usually prescribed.

Stoma bag The stoma care nurse will show your relative how to change the bag (see

below). There are different designs available.
Skin care Your relative will be shown how to wash and dry around the stoma and how to identify infection.
Diet Advice will be given on identifying and cutting out foods that cause problems.

Stoma bag

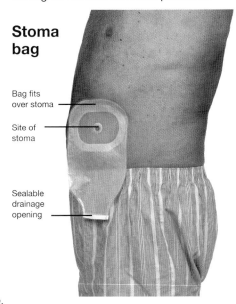

Bag fits over stoma

Site of stoma

Sealable drainage opening

CHANGING A STOMA BAG

The bag is usually changed twice a day. Allow your relative privacy, and ensure that he has everything he requires. For the procedure he will need a bowl of warm water, soap, a towel, a replacement bag and a disposal bag, which should be provided.
The normal procedure is as follows:

- the stoma bag is removed and placed in the disposal bag;
- the stoma and surrounding area is cleaned with warm water and soap, and dried thoroughly;
- the new bag is attached.

CHAPTER 11

HOME FROM HOSPITAL

Your role as a carer may begin when your relative is discharged from hospital. Before this happens, the hospital should ensure that you have all the resources you need to provide adequate aftercare.

AFTERCARE

Planning aftercare will be easier if you find out as much as possible about your relative's condition and the type of hospital treatment he has undergone. Contact your GP or Public Health Nurse for advice and support on community services. If you are caring for your relative full-time, you may need professional assistance or part-time help. The services of a day centre or respite may provide the psychological and physical care your relative needs, and can also offer you advice, support and some relief from your role.

REHABILITATION AND CONVALESCENCE

A major operation or illness may have a profound emotional effect on your relative, especially if he has restricted mobility and is dependent on others for the first time in his adult life. He may also take time to adjust to being back at home, particularly if he has been in hospital for a long period of time.

LEAVING HOSPITAL

You and your relative should be consulted from the outset by the hospital about arrangements for discharge; these arrangements may even begin before your relative goes into hospital or when he is admitted. As the main carer, you will be told when to collect him from hospital, how to care for him at home, how to administer medicines and what follow-up visits are required.

BEFORE YOUR RELATIVE IS DISCHARGED

Remember! Discharge should be planned for. Hospital staff should only discharge a patient when they are satisfied that there is someone to care for him at home. They should always consult the patient about this, and you, as the main carer. You will need to liaise with various members of staff, such as the nurse in charge, the social worker and the doctor, in planning your relative's discharge and aftercare.

QUESTIONS YOU SHOULD ASK THE HOSPITAL STAFF

Do not be afraid to ask questions about your relative's condition and the type of care he needs. Find out:
- what medicines he needs, how frequently they are required and how they should be administered;
- whether the medicines or the treatments have any side effects; if so, how these should be managed;
- how to carry out specific moving and handling manoeuvres, on your own or with help;
- how to cope should things go wrong.

PREPARATIONS THE HOSPITAL STAFF SHOULD MAKE

Before your relative leaves hospital, a member of staff will consult you, the main carer, and advise you when to collect him. They will also:
- inform the GP and Public Health Nurse of the discharge, and explain your relative's condition and likely needs;
- order the medicines for his immediate aftercare;
- arrange any specialised aftercare services, such as physiotherapy or occupational therapy;
- if necessary, arrange transport home;
- give you instructions regarding the aftercare and follow-up visits to the hospital and;
- advise your relative when he can return to work.

ENSURING YOUR NEEDS ARE MET

The welfare of your relative and yourself is paramount in the discharge procedure. You both have the right to complain if you are dissatisfied.

Hospital staff Firstly, speak to the nurse in charge or, if this fails, to the hospital manager.

Complaints procedure If you are still not satisfied, make a formal complaint according to the hospital's procedures.

Specialist help Seek help from the ward staff, your GP or local Community Health Centre on how to make a complaint. The Irish Patient's Association will also be able to advise you.

PREPARING THE HOME

Before your relative leaves hospital, you need to ensure that you have the necessary resources and skills to provide adequate care. You should find out from the nurse in charge or the doctor exactly what is required of you. Once you are satisfied that you can undertake the caring role, you can make preparations for your relative's return home.

PREPARING YOURSELF FOR CARING

Before you feel confident that you can provide adequate care, ask yourself the following questions:

- Do I fully understand why my relative was admitted to hospital and what treatments he received there?

- Am I physically and mentally capable of caring for my relative day and night?

- Who do I turn to in an emergency? Do I have the telephone numbers of the GP (on-call GP services) and Public Health Nurse?

- Do I have enough support from other people, such as a friend, relative or volunteer carer, where necessary, to help look after my relative?

- What effect will the caring role have on other members of my household?

- Is the home sufficiently equipped? For example, are special toilet facilities, or any special aids, such as a wheelchair, needed?

If you are unsure about any of the above, you should seek the advice of the nursing staff, your relative's GP and Public Health Nurse before agreeing to take on the caring role.

PRACTICAL ARRANGEMENTS AT HOME

Before your relative leaves hospital, you should make thorough preparations at home.

Preparing his room Ensure that your relative's bedroom is clean and comfortable and that it is not too hot or too cold. The layout of the room should be practical, with bedside items to hand.

Preparing a meal Have a light meal ready as he may be hungry, but bear in mind dietary restrictions.

Organising visitors Stagger visits from family and friends. Talk to your relative to see if he feels up to seeing people, bearing in mind that he may feel tired.

PROLONGED ILLNESSES

Caring for someone with a prolonged illness, such as cancer or kidney disease, can be particularly difficult. Your relative will require a lot of emotional support, especially if he is undergoing intensive treatment, such as chemotherapy or dialysis. The closer you are to someone, the more difficult it can be, so it is advisable to seek outside support.

Support groups The GP/Public Health Nurse can offer advice and support to the affected person, and the family on the range of organisations and support services available. A support group for carers, such as Carers Association, Caring For Carer's Irl., and Care Alliance Ireland may be able to put you and your relative in contact with others in a similar situation.

HOSPITAL OUT-PATIENT TREATMENTS

Many disorders can be treated in a hospital's outpatient department. Some day procedures are also required to investigate a condition to see if an operation is needed or to give treatment following an operation. Understanding the treatment will help you provide the best aftercare.

A GUIDE TO THE TREATMENTS AND AFTER-EFFECTS

TREATMENT	WHAT HAPPENS	AFTER-EFFECTS
BARIUM X-RAY	Barium is a white substance that shows up on an X-Ray. The patient swallows barium 'meal', which is then X-Rayed (as it progresses through the intestinal tract) to investigate the bowel and rectum. Barium may also be given as an enema.	White faeces may be passed. The patient may become constipated.
MRI SCAN	Magnetic Resonance Imaging (MRI) uses magnetic fields and radio waves to make detailed cross-sectional pictures of the head and body, which are translated by computer into high quality images. The patient will be asked to remove any metal objects and to lie as still as possible on a couch that moves through the scanner. He will hear instructions from the radiographer or nurse through headphones.	The scan is painless and there are no after-effects. It is noisy, but you will be offered earphones with music.
KEYHOLE SURGERY	For some conditions this is an alternative to major surgery. Tiny viewing instruments (scopes) are passed through small incisions in the body and then manipulated to examine and remove tissue and tumours. Typical procedures are treatment of some hernias and removing cartilage from a knee joint. It is also possible to remove the gall bladder in this way.	There will be some discomfort, but recuperation is swifter than concentrated surgery because the surgery is relatively minimal.

A GUIDE TO THE TREATMENTS AND AFTER-EFFECTS

TREATMENT	WHAT HAPPENS	AFTER-EFFECTS
CHEMOTHERAPY	The treatment of cancer may involve the injection of drugs through a vein in order to destroy abnormal cells. The first sessions usually take place in a cancer (oncology) unit; thereafter they may be continued in an outpatient department and sometimes at home. In other instances only tablets are required to be taken.	Vomiting and diarrhoea can leave the patient feeling weak and tired. Hair loss may occur.
RADIOTHERAPY	Radiotherapy is the treatment of cancer by radiation. High energy x-rays are used to destroy the tumour cells. The treatment can be given on a daily basis or over a number of weeks. It is a painless procedure. There are a number of steps involved in the preparation of the treatment. Radiotherapy may be used in conjunction with chemotherapy to treat some cancers.	The patient may feel tired during and after treatment. There may be side effects depending on the part of the body being treated. These are individual to each person.
KIDNEY DIALYSIS	A procedure designed to remove harmful toxic elements from the blood and excess fluid from the body as treatment for kidney failure.	Hunger, thirst and occasional confusion.
GASTROSCOPY	Long, flexible viewing instruments (approx. the diameter of an average adult ring finger) (gastroscopes) are passed through the mouth and used to investigate conditions of the stomach. A doctor views the stomach lining and takes biopsies to aid diagnosis.	Patients often complain of a sore throat and/or wind for a day or two after this procedure.
COLONOSCOPY	Long flexible viewing instruments are passed through the rectum and large intestine to investigate conditions of the bowel. A doctor views the lining and takes biopsies to aid diagnosis.	Patients often complain of abdominal soreness from trapped air for a day or two following the procedure.

DAY HOSPITALS

A Day Hospital provides outpatient services i.e. physiotherapy, occupational therapy and speech therapy. They are usually attached to General Hospitals. This service can be assessed from inpatient, outpatient or GP referral.

CONVALESCENCE

Recovery from an illness or operation may leave your relative immobile and restricted in what he is able to do. This often leads to reduced well-being, boredom, frustration and depression. You may be able to help by encouraging pastimes that will keep him busy, and his mind active. These activities can help him focus on regaining good health and maximum independence.

ACTIVITIES TO PROMOTE WELL-BEING

As soon as your relative is well enough, try to introduce activities that encourage a more positive state of mind. Music, hobbies, games and gentle exercise will greatly improve the later stages of recovery by providing mental and physical stimulation, offering a welcome diversion from immobility, and helping to boost confidence.

HOBBIES AND INTERESTS

As your relative begins to make progress, incorporate a hobby or interest into his daily routine with the use of appropriate aids. Equipment such as a kneeling frame, for example, allows a gardener to lower and raise himself with ease.

PLAYING GAMES

Playing cards or board games, and doing puzzles and jigsaws, are pastimes that you can enjoy together. These activities can help to keep your relative's mind alert, lift his spirits and encourage gentle motion of the upper body.

GENTLE EXERCISE

Encourage your relative to walk very short distances, then build on this according to his progress. If he is not able to walk, a short car ride will at least give him an opportunity to leave the house.

HANDICRAFTS

Crafts, such as knitting, painting and model-making, are absorbing for those who like working with their hands. These activities can be very therapeutic and are ideal for those whose mobility is restricted.

A range of music, exercise programmes and recreational activities may be available in your local area.

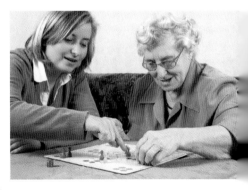

REHABILITATION

After your relative comes out of hospital, he may not be able to carry out some day-to-day tasks, such as having a bath or cooking for himself. You will need to assess the level of help he requires but, where possible, you should allow him to be independent. He may also have been prescribed treatment, such as physiotherapy, to take place at home, or at a day centre or hospital.

RE-ESTABLISHING A DAILY ROUTINE

You will need to establish a routine that will ease your relative back into home life and help him to regain his health. His daily timetable should be based on the information supplied by the hospital staff and on his individual needs. Bear in mind the following points, when working out a routine:

- how much rest he needs;
- what type of diet he requires;
- what he is physically capable of doing;
- what medication he takes;
- any specially devised aftercare programme, such as physiotherapy exercises;
- follow-up treatments at the hospital and check-up visits from his GP and Public Health Nurse.

PROMOTING WELL-BEING AND INDEPENDENCE

Once your relative is home, bear in mind his physical and emotional needs. He may be unable to carry out all the daily activities he undertook before going into hospital. He may feel insecure or even confused about being out of the routine of the hospital ward. Patience is required while he adjusts to the new location and a different way of doing things.

Rest Encourage him to take things slowly. He should rest for at least an hour in the afternoon, and catnap whenever he is tired.

Exercise If he is mobile, encourage him to take gentle exercise, even if it is only walking about indoors.

Companionship Try not to leave him alone for long periods, as he may feel isolated after being in a busy hospital ward. Although it is good for him to receive visitors, make sure he is ready for this. If possible, find time to talk to him about how he feels, and be encouraging and reassuring.

EMOTIONAL SUPPORT

Try to be sensitive to how your relative is feeling, particularly if he has experienced a major operation or an illness that required lengthy treatment. If he has had a life-changing operation or illness, he may benefit from outside support, such as counselling, to overcome any distress.

Gathering information Find out as much as you can from the hospital staff about your relative's illness and the likely effects of the treatment he has recently undergone.

Seeking support Various support groups have been established to help people care for specific conditions. Ask your GP or Public Health Nurse to put you in touch with one for help and advice, or telephone the relevant organisation directly for information.

TREATMENTS AND THERAPIES

Rehabilitation means restoring an individual to normal function after a disease or injury. This process can take a long time and may require your relative to undergo regular treatments and therapies:

- as part of his treatment, your relative may be shown exercises that he can carry out himself;
- as the main carer, you may be taught simple techniques that you can regularly administer at home;
- a qualified therapist might visit your home to treat your relative;
- your relative may go for treatment at a day centre, which might also be linked to a hospital.

DAY CENTRES

Day centres allow your relative to meet people who have similar needs, and give you, the carer, the chance to have a break. They also cater for people who require assistance in some daily activity such as preparing food, bathing or washing clothes.

THE RANGE OF THERAPIES

Following a thorough assessment of your relative's condition, the most effective treatment is prescribed.

Physiotherapy This is a combination of exercises prescribed by a physiotherapist for the patient's individual needs. The exercises are used to strengthen and heal parts of the body in conjunction with heat treatments or ultrasound, for example.

Hydrotherapy These are exercise sessions that take place in a swimming pool. Water reduces the pull of gravity on the injured part of the body, making movement easier and so reducing pain.

Occupational therapy This form of therapy helps a person to relearn everyday skills that have been lost as a result of illness or injury, such as dressing, bathing and preparing meals. It is particularly useful for stroke patients or for those who are otherwise disabled.

Speech therapy This range of exercises is designed to help someone overcome a language, speech or swallowing difficulties.

PHYSIOTHERAPY AT HOME

A physiotherapist will demonstrate techniques to help your relative strengthen his limbs and improve dexterity.

Hand therapy Special items, such as soft balls, can be manipulated by hand to improve dexterity and strengthen wrist and hand movement.

Limb therapy This is effective for someone who has restricted movement. A common exercise may require you, the carer, to hold the limb (at the wrist and elbow, or ankle and knee) and move it upwards, exercising all the joints without pushing beyond the natural movement of the limb.

Physiotherapy exercises You can help your relative by carrying out gentle limb therapy.

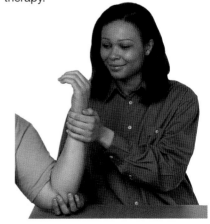

CHAPTER 12

CARE SKILLS

Part of your role may involve caring for your relative while she has a long or short-term illness. As with all aspects of caring, looking after an ill person at home requires common sense. Your main aims are to make sure that your relative is comfortable and, where possible, to help in alleviating any painful or distressing symptoms. For example, if she can't get out of bed, something as simple as keeping the room clean and well-ventilated may help to make her feel better or if, for example, she has a condition that causes breathing difficulties, you may be able to help by making sure that she is in a comfortable position.

PRACTICAL SKILLS

The pages that follow give you a basic understanding of the practical skills you need to look after someone who is ill: how to take someone's temperature and measure her pulse rate, how to relieve uncomfortable symptoms and what information to record and pass on to the doctor. There is also a guide to the type of medication that is likely to be prescribed. If you are unable to deal with any aspect of this type of caring, are concerned about your relative's symptoms, or are unclear on any aspects of her medication, always seek the advice of a healthcare professional, such as a GP or Public Health Nurse.

TEMPERATURE CHANGES

A healthy body maintains a constant temperature of between 36-37°C (96.8-98.6°F) by achieving a balance between the heat it produces and the heat it loses. If this balance is disturbed, a body temperature outside the normal range will result. This is often a sign of illness, so you will need to seek medical help and, in the meantime, try to alleviate any symptoms.

RECOGNISING AN ABNORMAL TEMPERATURE

If the body temperature falls below 36°C (96.8°F) or rises above 37°C (98.6°F), there may be clear signs. Pulse and breathing rates may also indicate an abnormal temperature.

SIGNS OF A VERY LOW TEMPERATURE

The person will feel cold and may be:
• shivering • pale • confused

SIGNS OF A HIGH TEMPERATURE

The person will feel hot and may:
• have flushed cheeks
• be sweating
• be shivering

TAKING A TEMPERATURE

There are a range of aids for taking the temperature, always follow the manufacturers guidelines on how and where it should be taken.

The site used for taking the temperature depends on the device available. Sites include the forehead, ear, mouth (oral) and under the arm (axilla). To ensure an accurate temperature reading, the thermometer needs close body contact for the time recommended by the manufacturer. Remember, oral temperature is higher than the axilla temperature. Make sure to practice good infection control.

Low temperature A drop in temperature below 35°C (95°F) (hypothermia) occurs when the body loses more heat than it can produce. This can occur outdoors in very cold weather conditions, and indoors if preventive measures are not taken.

High temperature This is part of the body's natural defence mechanism for fighting infection. The increase in temperature above 37°C (98.6°F) (pyrexia), helps to destroy many bacteria and viruses.

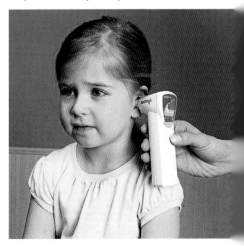

THERMOMETERS

There are now many different devices available for measuring temperature.

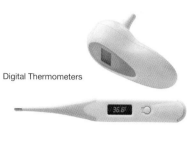

Digital Thermometers

- Digital and Infra Red thermometers measures the temperature, which is then displayed digitally in a window

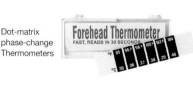

Dot-matrix phase-change Thermometers

- Dot-matrix phase-change thermometers are plastic strips, which change colour as they heat up, giving a temperature reading.

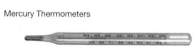

Mercury Thermometers

- Mercury thermometers indicate the temperature by means of a mercury level. They are now almost obsolete because of the difficulty of reading and the danger of mercury spilling out if the glass breaks.

Many thermometers have probe covers, which are discarded after each use, whereas others need to be disinfected with cleaning agents - follow the manufacturer's recommendations.

A GUIDE TO TEMPERATURE
- 36 - 37°C (96.8 - 98.6°F) = normal
- above 37°C (98.6°F) = fever
- below 35°C (95°F) = hypothermia

WHEN NOT TO USE THE MOUTH

Taking the temperature by mouth is not safe or effective if someone:
- is unconscious;
- is confused or mentally impaired;
- is a baby, or a child aged under six;
- is suffering from a jaw injury;
- is susceptible to convulsions;
- has a cough or blocked nose;
- has recently had a hot or cold drink.

TAKING A TEMPERATURE UNDER THE ARMPIT

1 Rinse the thermometer in cold water and dry it with a clean cloth. If you are using a digital thermometer, switch it on.

2 Make sure the thermometer and the skin under the armpit are dry. Ask the person to keep still.

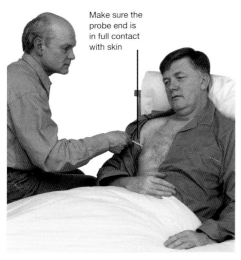

Make sure the probe end is in full contact with skin

3 Place the thermometer in the person's armpit and ask him to fold his forearm across his chest.

4 Leave the thermometer in place for two minutes or until it bleeps.

5 Record the temperature by noting the reading.

6 A digital thermometer needs to be switched off. Wipe the thermometer clean and return it to its case.

BREATHING AND PULSE RATES

While taking a temperature, you should check your relative's breathing and pulse rates as an increase or decrease in these can also indicate a temperature change. The information can then be recorded and given to the GP, along with the temperature reading.

Monitor breathing At rest, a person breathes in and out (one respiration) about 16 times per minute. Anything above or below this may accompany a high or low temperature. Count your relative's breaths per minute and note your findings for the GP. To get a more accurate measure, do not tell him that you are monitoring his breathing.

Check the pulse The pulse is the 'wave' that courses through the body each time the heart pumps blood into the circulatory system. The normal pulse rate for an adult at rest is between 60-80 beats per minute; anything above or below this level, and any change in the strength of the pulse, may accompany a high or low temperature.

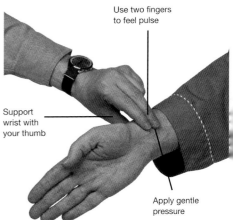

Use two fingers to feel pulse

Support wrist with your thumb

Apply gentle pressure

How to take a pulse Place your fingertips in the hollow just above the wrist creases at the base of the thumb. Count the beats for one minute and record the figure. Try to judge the strength of the pulse as well as the rhythm.

DEALING WITH A HIGH TEMPERATURE

A high temperature is usually the result of an infection, and may, therefore, be impossible to prevent and difficult to control at times.

TREATING A HIGH TEMPERATURE

Your aims are to try to lower the temperature and make your relative comfortable. Call the GP if a high temperature persists or you are worried.

Offer the chance to freshen up Ask your relative if he would like a wash, and a change of clothes and bed linen.

Monitor room temperature Ensure that the room is adequately ventilated. You can use a fan, but do not overchill.

Provide fluids and food Give him plenty of cold drinks, and offer frequent mouthwashes. Loss of fluid may cause appetite loss and sluggish bowel movements, so provide light meals only.

Medication Is available to lower the temperature. Consult your pharmacist or GP.

Cool with water Sponge your relative all over with tepid water, but do not let him get too cold. Gently dry him afterwards. Alternatively, apply a cool compress to his forehead.

Applying a compress

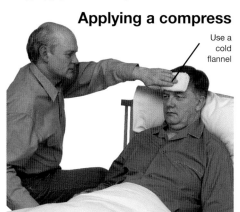

Use a cold flannel

DEALING WITH A LOW TEMPERATURE

Hypothermia can occur when the body temperature drops below 35°C (95°F) and if the surrounding temperature is especially cold. Those most at risk are elderly, immobile and ill people.

TREATING HYPOTHERMIA

Hypothermia is a life-threatening condition, so urgent medical help should always be sought. An elderly person should be rewarmed gradually.

PREVENTING HYPOTHERMIA

Take steps to prevent your relative from getting hypothermia.

Regulate room temperature The temperature drops at night, so ensure that the bedroom is kept at around 18°C (64.4°F). Seek advice on financial allowances for heating bills for someone with a limited income.

Provide sufficient food and drink Hot food and drink, and regular meals, are essential.

Provide effective clothing Several layers of light clothing are more effective than one thick layer. Gloves and socks help to keep extremities such as fingers and toes warm. Remember a lot of body heat is lost through the head so wear a hat even indoors, when it is cold.

Encourage movement Exercise helps the circulation of blood. A few minutes walking around the room will help if your relative is able to do so.

BLOOD PRESSURE

Blood pressure is the pressure exerted against the blood vessel walls by the blood as it flows through them. It is usually measured at the brachial artery, at the crease of the elbow.

Blood pressure is measured with an instrument called a sphygmomanometer. First, a cuff is placed around the patient's arm and inflated with a pump until the circulation is cut off. A small valve slowly deflates the cuff. The blood pressure is measured using a stethoscope placed over the patient's arm to listen for the sound of blood flow to return through the arteries. This first sound is the systolic blood pressure; this is when the heart is contracting and pumping blood around the blood vessels. Once the pulse fades it indicates the diastolic pressure, the blood pressure of your heart at rest between beats.

patient as required, sitting or lying. Ensure the sphygmomanometer is positioned at heart level. With the palm of the hand facing upwards, apply the cuff of the sphygmomanometer snugly around the arm. Locate the radial pulse and inflate the cuff until the radial pulse can no longer be felt. Place the bell of the stethoscope over the brachial artery. Place the ear pieces in your ears, and slowly deflate the cuff by releasing the control valve. Record both the Systolic Pressure and Diastolic Pressure. Remove the equipment and clean after use. Use alcohol wipes to clean the stethoscope. Clean the Sphygmomanometer, and store safely.

MANUAL BLOOD PRESSURE

Assemble the required equipment. Explain the procedure to the patient. Position the

DIGITAL BLOOD PRESSURE

Assemble the required equipment. Explain the procedure to the patient. Position the patient as required, sitting or lying. Switch on the monitor. Remove any restrictive clothing. The machine can be used once the heart symbol is displayed. Fit the cuff comfortably around the left upper arm with the air tube towards the wrist. Ensure the cuff is level with the heart. Press the start button to the inflate cuff. Ask the patient to sit still and not to talk during the process. Record the Blood Pressure and Pulse displayed. Turn off the machine once deflated, and store safely.

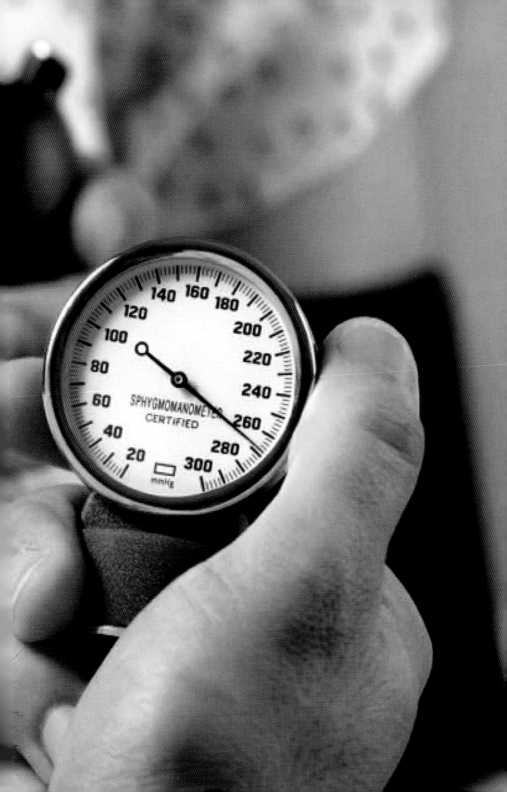

BREATHING DIFFICULTIES

If the person you are caring for experiences difficulty breathing, you should seek medical advice immediately. Breathlessness may be a symptom of a short-term illness, such as the flu, but it could also result from a lung condition, such as asthma, or even a heart problem. Treatments range from self-help remedies to the use of specialist equipment.

ALLEVIATING BREATHING DIFFICULTIES

Breathing difficulties can be prevented or minimised by considering environmental factors, and by the person assuming the most comfortable and effective posture to ease breathing.

ENVIRONMENT

A room's atmosphere may aggravate your relative's breathing difficulties. Try to establish whether there are any specific factors that appear to improve or worsen the condition and, if possible, make changes to alleviate the problem.

Ventilate rooms Hot rooms, especially those that are centrally heated, can aggravate respiratory problems. You can help by making sure that:
• rooms are adequately ventilated;
• the heating is not too high;
• the atmosphere is not too dry (a bowl of water placed in the room can increase humidity).

Pinpoint allergies There may be contributing factors to your relative's condition. You can help by:
• keeping known allergens, such as animal fur or feather pillows, away;
• keeping the environment as clean and dust-free as possible.

Encourage outdoor activities
Being outdoors may help to alleviate the problem. Encourage your relative to:
• go for walks in pollution-free areas;
• sit in the garden, if the weather allows.

POSTURE

There are various positions that a person can assume whether in bed or in a chair that can make breathing easier. Your relative will probably know which position is most comfortable, so always listen to him. The positions include:
• sitting in an upright chair, supported by pillows or a backrest;
• sitting upright in a bed with pillows or a specially designed backrest;
• leaning forwards with arms supported on a chair or a stool, for temporary relief.

Leaning forwards to aid breathing

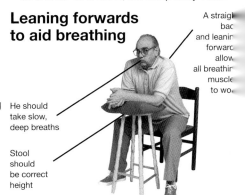

A straigh
bac
and leanir
forwarc
allow
all breathir
muscle
to wo

He should
take slow,
deep breaths

Stool
should
be correct
height

MEDICATION FOR BREATHING DIFFICULTIES

Medication can vary from antibiotics for chest infections, to inhalers and oxygen for more long-term breathing difficulties.

PRESCRIBED INHALERS

Someone with a breathing difficulty, such as asthma, may be prescribed an inhaler and shown how to use it; the device enables medication to be inhaled directly into the lungs. Make sure an inhaler and a refill are always readily available and in date. There are different types.

Preventer inhaler This is usually brown or white. A sufferer uses it regularly to prevent an attack.

Reliever inhaler This type of inhaler is usually blue. It is used during an attack to open the airways.

Spacer This device has a mouthpiece at one end and a hole for the inhaler at the other end. The inhaler is inserted into the spacer and the medication is squirted into it before being breathed in through the mouthpiece. These are often used to enable a child, elderly person or someone who is weak to inhale the medication more effectively.

Nebuliser This is a small machine that provides a larger dose of medication than an inhaler. It is only used when breathing difficulties are severe.

Using an inhaler

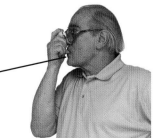

As he breathes in, medication is released

STEAM INHALATION

A simple home remedy for loosening phlegm and easing coughing is to add an inhalant to steaming hot water. The person then inhales the steam. Inhalation can be an effective treatment for colds, flu and mild bronchitis. Ask your pharmacist to recommend an inhalant.

Method Add the inhalant to a bowl of hot water, following the instructions on the bottle. Ask the person to sit down and place his face directly over the bowl. Make sure that:
• the water is not boiling hot;
• his face is not too close to the water.
Place a towel over his head, large enough to cover his head and the bowl. Advise him to inhale for up to ten minutes, and stay with him throughout.

PHYSIOTHERAPY

Breathlessness may be treated with physiotherapy. Chest physiotherapy, postural drainage and breathing techniques are simple treatments that can be carried out at home. In an illness such as cystic fibrosis, these can help to minimise infection by enabling the lungs to keep clear of the sticky mucus brought on by the condition. After surgery, especially when the chest cavity has been opened, breathing exercises can help the person to regain normal breathing patterns. Whatever the condition, a physiotherapist will train you in the techniques that are suitable for your relative's age and illness. Treatment may be daily, or more often for serious conditions.

GIVING OXYGEN

Oxygen may be prescribed for chronic chest or heart complaints.

For intermittent use Oxygen is supplied by a cylinder in the home and given via a mask.

For continuous use Equipment may be installed in the home to provide a continuous supply of oxygen to the person.

To aid mobility In addition to a large cylinder, the person may be given a portable cylinder, enabling her to walk around, climb stairs and leave the house and still receive oxygen.

Oxygen cyclinder

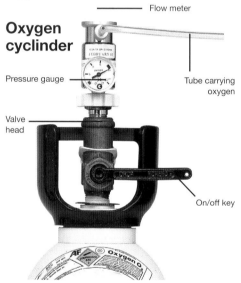

Flow meter

Pressure gauge

Tube carrying oxygen

Valve head

On/off key

OXYGEN PRECAUTIONS

Always follow instructions carefully:
• only give oxygen at the rate prescribed;
• monitor oxygen level;
• check level of water in any humidifier;
• keep cylinders away from fires, naked flames, electrical toys, grease and oil;
• do not smoke near oxygen cylinders;
• always keep spare supplies;
• store cylinders in a cool place.

GIVING OXYGEN BY MASK

1 Before giving oxygen, read the pressure gauge to check how much oxygen the cylinder contains.

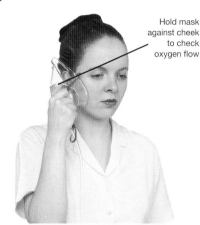

Hold mask against cheek to check oxygen flow

2 Connect the tube of the mask to the cylinder, as instructed. Use the key to open the cylinder valve and adjust the rate of flow of oxygen according to the instructions. Check that the oxygen is flowing by holding the mask near to your cheek.

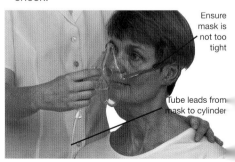

Ensure mask is not too tight

Tube leads from mask to cylinder

3 Arrange the mask over the person's nose and mouth. Record the amount of oxygen given in litres per minute. You may be provided with a mask through which a fixed percentage of oxygen is delivered.

MEDICATION

There are two categories of medication: those that require a doctor's prescription and those that do not. You should have an understanding of why your relative needs to take any medication, and be aware of potential side effects. Your main aims are to make sure medication is taken correctly and, wherever possible, allow your relative to take it by himself.

MEDICATION GUIDELINES

When assisting with medication, follow the four basic rules:
• right person
• right medicine
• right amount
• right time

PRESCRIBED MEDICATION

Follow the GP's instructions and always read the label and accompanying leaflets. Contact the GP's surgery or the pharmacist for advice if necessary.

OVER-THE-COUNTER MEDICATION

There has been a huge increase in the availability of over-the-counter drugs that do not require a prescription. These are available at supermarkets and local shops, as well as at chemists. If your relative is already on medication, or you have any doubts about the drugs you are buying, you should always seek the advice of a pharmacist or GP.

SIDE EFFECTS OF MEDICATION

Read the leaflet supplied with the medication or check with the GP and the pharmacist about any side effects.

Drowsiness The person will be advised not to drink alcohol, drive or operate machinery.

Diet The GP or the pharmacist should advise if any dietary restrictions need to be observed.

Adverse reactions Side effects, such as diarrhoea, vomiting, dizziness, skin rashes and any other unexpected problems should be reported to the GP.

DO'S & DON'TS

Do wash your hands before and after giving medication.

Do check the expiry date of medication.

Do store medication in a safe place and where necessary in a child-proof container.

Do follow storage instructions.

Do dispose of needles and syringes correctly.

Do return unwanted medication to a pharmacist for disposal.

Don't give the medication if it has changed colour or has turned cloudy.

Don't give the medication if you are unable to read the label.

Don't store different pills in one bottle.

Don't decant from one bottle into another.

TYPES OF MEDICATION

Liquids Always shake the bottle to mix the constituents thoroughly. Follow the instructions on the bottle and use the correct size of measuring spoon. Don't use the medicine if it has changed colour or turned cloudy.

Tablets These can be crushed and mixed with honey or jam, unless there are dietary restrictions. Eneric coated tablets and those that have a shiny shell should be swallowed whole, if possible, with a drink.

Capsules These should not be broken open as they are designed to dissolve slowly in the stomach. They are easier to swallow if placed at the back of the tongue and taken with a drink.

Powders These can be stirred and dissolved in liquids or foods but check that no dietary restrictions apply.

Sup positories and pessaries
Suppositories are inserted into the rectum; pessaries into the vagina. The person should insert these according to medical instruction. Do not administer them yourself unless properly instructed.

Creams/lotions Some lotions and creams contain powerful drugs, such as steroids. Always follow the instructions on the tube or bottle. It is advisable to wear latex gloves when applying some creams and lotions. Always wash hands before and after.

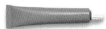

Inhalers These enable a person to inhale drugs to alleviate breathing difficulties. Colour coding enables you to differentiate between the different types.

Needles/Pens A person who needs regular medication by injection is usually taught how to do this himself. Ensure that the dosage is correct and that needles/pens are disposed of safely.

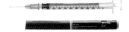

MONITORING DOSAGE

The person you are caring for may be on more than one type of medication, and knowing when to take each one can be confusing. To help, a pharmacist can supply the medication in a way that makes it easy to monitor dosage. Compartmentalised cassettes or blister packs can be used so that the person can see at a glance which medication to take and when to take it. Each compartment or pack is labelled with the day and the time the named dose is to be taken.

Advantages This system enables you to:
• monitor dosages of medication, while allowing your relative to be independent;
• minimise the risk of conflicting medications being taken together;
• in an emergency, provide instant information about which medication the person has taken.

ADMINISTERING EYE, NOSE AND EAR DROPS

Medications for the eye, nose and ear usually come in the form of drops. These are sterile and should always be used before the expiry date on the package. If only one eye or ear is affected, make sure that you apply drops to the correct side, as it can be dangerous to use medication on healthy organs. When applying eye drops, do not allow the dropper to come into contact with the eye as this can often cause infection to spread. Wash the dropper should it become contaminated. It is common for steroids or drugs such as antibiotics and antihistamines to be given in eye, nose or ear drop form.

APPLYING EYE DROPS

1 Stand behind the person. Ask him to lean his head back against you and look up.

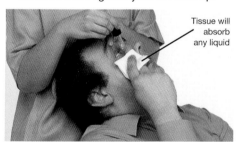

Tissue will absorb any liquid

2 Give him a tissue to hold against his cheek. Gently pull back the upper eyelid. Squeeze the correct dosage into the space between the lower eyelid and the eyeball, near to the inside corner of the eye.

3 The person will automatically close his eye. Ask him to blink a couple of times. This disperses the eye drop over the whole surface of the eye.

APPLYING NASAL DROPS

1 Ask the person to blow his nose so that any blockage is cleared before applying the drops.

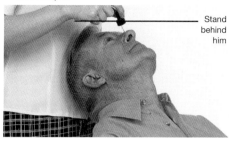

Stand behind him

2 Ask him to tilt his head as far back as possible. Insert the tip of the dropper just inside the nostril and squeeze out the correct dosage. Repeat this procedure for the other nostril.

3 Ask him to sniff to disperse the drops within the nasal cavity. Advise him to stay in the same position for a short while and to refrain from blowing his nose for at least 20 minutes.

APPLYING EAR DROPS

1 Ask the person to tilt her head so that the affected ear is uppermost.

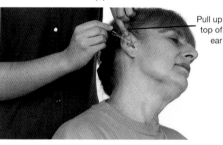

Pull up top of ear

2 Grip top of the ear. Hold the dropper just above the opening. Allow the drops to trickle into the ear canal.

3 Ask the person to keep her head still, in the same position, for a few minutes.

4 Place a piece of cotton wool just over the opening to the ear. Under no circumstances should the cotton wool be pushed into the ear canal.

WOUND CARE

A wound is a break in the skin and may be the result of an injury, disease or an operation. The kind of care needed depends on the size and severity of the wound. Professional help should be sought to carry out a full assessment. Wounds due to an operation or conditions such as varicose ulcers may require regular aftercare, and a Public Health Nurse will usually carry this out.

THE MAIN AIMS WHEN DRESSING A WOUND ARE:
- To prevent bacteria entering the wound and;
- To hasten healing and alleviate pain.

PREVENTING INFECTION
To prevent the wound becoming infected always:
- Wash your hands before treatment;
- Wear sterile latex gloves if possible;
- Clean the area so that dirt is washed away;
- Cover the wound with a dressing, preferably sterile;
- Dry the surrounding skin with a clean towel;
- Secure dressings properly and keep them dry;
- Dispose of used dressings and gloves and;
- It is a good idea to keep a basic first aid kit, which includes sterile dressings.

AN INFECTED WOUND
Seek medical advice if the wound begins to ooze and the skin around the wound becomes red, there is swelling, discomfort or the person complains of feeling hot or being in pain.

AIDING THE HEALING PROCESS
Babies and children heal much more rapidly than someone who is unwell or elderly.

Those with an underlying condition that requires drugs such as steroids, or others that suppress their immunity, may heal less quickly.

What the body requires In order for a wound to heal a person needs to be physically healthy and well nourished. If a wound fails to heal it may be because of an underlying condition, such as anaemia, the advice of a healthcare professional such as a GP or Public Health Nurse should be sought.

THE HEALING PROCESS
When any part of the body has been damaged as a result of, for example a cut or pressure sore, tissues adjacent to the injured area will begin to repair the damage. If tissue has been lost, as occurs with a burn or an abscess, for example, or if the affected area has been contaminated in any way, it will take longer to heal itself.

The body repairs the damaged area in the following way:
- The wound bleeds, the blood clots, then dries to form a scab;
- White blood cells begin to destroy and remove dead and damaged tissue;
- Cells grow rapidly in the clotted blood and
- Firm, fibrous tissues form across the wound and may become a scar.

CHAPTER 13

PALLIATIVE CARE

Palliative care is the active total care of patients whose condition is incurable.
The aim of palliative care is to achieve the best quality of life for patients and
their families. It includes control of pain, ease of symptoms of the illness, and
social, spiritual and psychological help leading to a peaceful and dignified death.
Palliative care offers a support system to help the patient live as actively as
possible until death, and also helps the family cope during the patient's illness
and death. Many people prefer to die at home in familiar surroundings and in the
company of their families. The Palliative Care Team, GP, Public Health Nurse and
voluntary agencies can provide specialist help and support.

CLOSE RELATIONSHIPS

Although caring for someone who is dying is stressful and upsetting, it can also be a
very positive experience for both the person who is dying and their carers. It may reunite
a family, forge friendships and provide an opportunity to express affection. Close
relationships between the carer and the family and friends are likely to continue after
the death, and can be a great source of comfort and support to those who are grieving.

FACING DEATH

Finding out that someone is going to die brings with it a wide range of emotions. Your dying relative may fear death, pain or simply the unknown. You may have fears about seeing someone who is close to you suffer, and you may worry about being left alone once he has died. These fears are understandable; talking about them openly may help you begin to cope.

WHEN THE NEWS IS BROKEN

You may be one of the first people to be informed that your relative is terminally ill, but it is the responsibility of the healthcare professional, not you, to inform him of this. You will, however, need to be prepared for how you handle this delicate subject.

Be informed If possible, try to be present when your relative receives the news: by listening and learning about his condition you may be able to provide comfort and support later.

Be honest If your relative asks you to expand on any detail, try to tell the truth as sensitively as possible. If there are any questions you cannot answer, seek the advice of a healthcare professional.

Be discreet Your relative may not wish to discuss death, or may even refuse to believe he is dying. If you need to talk about it, discuss the issue with the rest of the family or with an outsider, such as the GP.

THE IMPORTANCE OF COMMUNICATION

As death approaches, it is important that the dying person is encouraged to share his feelings.

Talking Do not be put off if he is unable to speak; listening to you talking can be very soothing.

Listening If he is able to express his wishes and sentiments, listen patiently and carefully; this is one of the most important things you can do for him.

Writing If he finds it difficult to talk, suggest that he writes down his feelings.

Touching Hold his hand; this can soothe anxieties and communicate reassurance and affection.

Counselling Your relative may benefit from talking to someone outside her family and close friends, such as a professional counsellor.

DO'S & DON'TS

The quality of care you provide will improve if you also look after your own needs.

Do acknowledge your own grief. It is a sign of human strength, not human failing.

Do turn to healthcare professionals for their support, and take advantage of their experience and expertise.

Do seek the help of volunteer carers.

Don't feel guilty if you are angry or frightened that your relative is dying. These emotions are natural, but try confiding in others rather than depressing your relative.

Don't bottle up your emotions as this may create even more stress.

Don't regard yourself as useless. You are providing essential support in a difficult time of need.

STAGES OF GRIEF

After the initial shock of learning that someone is terminally ill, there are various emotions and stages of grief that may affect those concerned. It can be an unsettling time; one moment you may be deeply emotional, the next you may feel numb. You will be able to cope better, and support your relative more effectively, if you are as open as possible about your feelings.

STAGES OF GRIEF

D : DENIAL
It's not happening
A : ANGER
Very annoyed and angry
- why me/us/him/her
B : BARGAINING
If you do this/that, it won't happen
D : DEPRESSION
Down in the dumps
A : ACCEPTANCE
OK, now what?

MAKING PATIENT COMFORTABLE

- Total nursing care
- Make comfortable
- Respectful
- Tend to any special needs and requests
- **NB: Dignity**
- Be aware of specific religious beliefs/customs

CARERS FEELINGS

When caring for someone who is dying, it's most important to be aware of your own feelings, for example.
- Recent bereavement
- Unresolved grief reaction
- Specific circumstances may be very similar to those close to yourself

In caring for someone else, it should not be used to resolve your own problem. Remember your sole role here is Carer. It is important to seek support for yourself if necessary.

HELP FROM OTHER AGENCIES

- GP
- Public Health Nurse
- Home Help
- Hospice Home Care Team
- Occupational Therapist - i.e. equipment

PRACTICAL CARE

When you are caring for a dying relative, one of your main aims will be to give him the best quality of life possible. This means making sure that he is comfortable, free of pain and, to alleviate boredom and depression, has enough to keep him occupied. Always try to respect your relative's wishes and encourage him to be as independent as possible.

COMFORTABLE SURROUNDINGS

If your relative is confined to bed or to the house, personal space will be extremely important to him. You can help by trying to make him feel comfortable and in control of his surroundings.

THE ROOM

For your relative's comfort, make sure his surroundings are kept clean and pleasant.
Ventilate the room A stuffy room can be unpleasant: open the windows, but avoid creating a draught.
Find the right level of light Arrange the curtains so that as much or as little light comes into the room to suit your relative's needs.
Make the room look pleasant Fresh flowers will add colour and fragrance, and liven up the room. Potpourri and scented candles may freshen the air.

VISITORS

Before encouraging friends or relatives to visit, make sure your relative wants to see them. Ideally, visits should be restricted to people with whom your relative feels comfortable. Do not be afraid to cancel visits if you feel that he is unable to cope. Remember, also, that too many visitors may put a strain on you, as the carer.

Monitor the length of visits Short, frequent visits are better than irregular, drawn-out ones that may be exhausting for your relative.
Restrict numbers of visitors One or two visitors at a time may be less overwhelming than large groups.
Prepare visitors Try to prepare visitors for your relative's appearance and attitude. They may find it awkward or feel shocked or upset if he is physically different or very depressed.

PROFESSIONAL SUPPORT

You may feel unable to give enough time to your relative, offer adequate care or cope with the many demands on your own. In this situation, you may need to seek part or full-time professional help. Consult the GP and Public Health Nurse for advice and information on what help is available.
Think ahead Anticipate when you might need the extra help and try to make the necessary arrangements before you find yourself in a crisis situation.
Seek short-term help Some local health authorities and charities have agencies that provide short-term care.
Seek full-time help Hospices, nursing homes or specialist organisations provide care for the terminally ill, and help and advise those looking after the person.

DAILY CARE

Encourage your relative to eat and drink, keep clean and generally look after himself. Accept, however, that he may not want to do so. Inform the GP if your relative has any uncomfortable symptoms, such as bowel problems, vomiting or pressure sores.

EATING AND DRINKING

Eating meals He may prefer small, appetising snacks at frequent intervals rather than three large meals a day. Make a note of any changes in appetite, and report them to the healthcare professional.

Drinking fluids Even if your relative does not wish to eat, encourage him to drink plenty of fluids.

PERSONAL HYGIENE AND APPEARANCE

Washing Encourage your relative to wash and bathe for his personal comfort and dignity. If confined to bed, he may require a bed bath.

Personal grooming You can help by offering to wash and brush your relative's hair and cut his fingernails and toenails. A man may feel better if he has had a shave, and a woman may require assistance with applying make-up, especially when visitors are expected.

Getting dressed Unless your relative is confined to bed, it is not necessary for him to stay in nightwear. Encourage him to get dressed, as this can give dignity and bolster confidence.

Using the toilet Encourage your relative to get out of bed to use the toilet. If he cannot, obtain toilet aids that allow maximum independence.

LIVING LIFE TO THE FULL

Mobility If your relative is able, he should be encouraged to be mobile, even if this only means getting out of bed to sit in a chair.

Hobbies If he is physically able, try to stimulate interest in pastimes that you know he enjoys. This may give pleasure, and encouragement to live the remainder of his life to the full.

HELPING TO MINIMISE PAIN

A dying person's greatest fear may be the prospect of coping with pain.

Reassure your relative You can reassure your relative that from the time of diagnosis, and throughout his care, he will be given medicines to minimise pain.

Act promptly Should he suffer pain at any time, inform a healthcare professional so that the situation can be rectified as soon as possible.

Find out about specialist equipment The use of specialist equipment will be explained to you, and administered under the supervision of a healthcare professional. For example, a pain relieving device such as a TENS (Transcutaneous Electrical Nerve Stimulator) may be recommended, or syringe pumps may be used to administer pain-relieving drugs. Speak to the GP about what is suitable.

Consider alternative therapies Your relative may prefer to try techniques such as reflexology, aromatherapy and visualisation.

TOWARDS THE END OF LIFE

One of the most delicate areas you may have to discuss with your relative is their funeral, but it is important not to force the issue. If they do want to talk about it, ask if they have preferences regarding the following:

MAKING ARRANGEMENTS IN ADVANCE

- Whether they wish to be buried or cremated;
- Any particular hymns or readings they may want at the memorial service;
- The type of headstone or memorial and inscription they would like;
- Where they want the ashes to be scattered;
- If the person carries a donor card.

FIND OUT IMPORTANT INFORMATION

Find out the names, addresses and telephone numbers of people who should be notified of the death, and locate the following documents:

- The will;
- Medical card;
- Birth and marriage certificates;
- Insurance, pension or other policies;
- Bank details.

WHAT DO I DO WHEN SOMEONE HAS DIED?

- Call the General Practitioner (GP): When he/she arrives, advise the GP of the approximate time and nature of the death. If the GP has attended within 28 days prior to death, the GP can issue the 'Medical Certificate of the Cause of Death'. This Certificate means that you are legally entitled to proceed with making funeral arrangements.
- The official Death Certificate is not required for making funeral arrangements. Since December 2005, the next-of-kin must now register a death within three months.
- Where the death is sudden, unexpected, following an accident, the Coroner for the district/county will become involved.
- Inform the Family: close members of the family may wish to spend some time alone with the person before the Funeral Directors' personnel remove the body.
- Lay the body flat face upwards. Remove the pillows, duvet and blankets. Do not worry or become over upset about straightening the body or limbs. Switch off any heater that may be on in the room. The body will assume the same temperature as its surroundings.
- Call the chosen 'Funeral Director'. They will arrange to remove the body to their preparation room where the preservation and care/dressing of the body will take place. The body may then be returned to the location of your choice e.g. family home, nursing home or funeral home.
- Inform the relevant insurance companies
- When practical, the Department of Social & Family Affairs should be informed if the

deceased was in receipt of a Social
Welfare Payment e.g. Old Age Pension.

ARRANGING THE FUNERAL

If you discussed the funeral with your
relative before he/she died, you may already
know what kind of service is required. The
funeral director will:
- Contact the place of burial or cremation;
- Discuss the type of service you require
  and any other arrangements necessary,
  for example, death notice in newspaper;
- Arrange a suitable date and time for the
  service.

YOU WILL NEED TO

- Notify friends and relatives of the date
  and venue;
- Organise flowers, if required, for the
  service;
- Organise a venue for a post funeral
  gathering.

HELP WITH FUNERAL COSTS

- It may be possible to claim a
  Bereavement Grant depending on
  your circumstances.

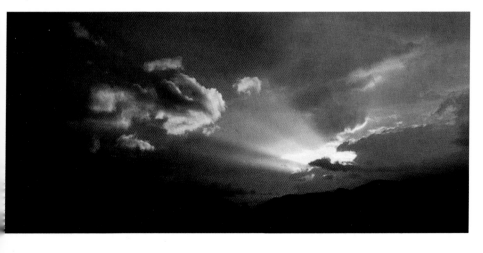

ROLE OF THE VOLUNTEER CARER

The demands on you as a volunteer carer outside the family circle will be great at this time. Family members and friends of the person who is dying may need you as much as, if not more than, the person in your care, and this can be particularly stressful. To help you cope with the demands and strains of your role, bear in mind what people will expect of you during this time.

COMPLEMENTARY CARE

Your responsibility as a carer outside the family circle is to complement, not dominate, the care regime. Try to achieve a balance between supporting the needs of the person and those who are close to him. Allow family and friends to be involved in his care and respect confidentiality.

ESSENTIAL QUALITIES OF THE CARER

As a volunteer carer, you will need to be a source of strength and support at all times; not only to the person in your care, but also to the dying person's close family and friends.

Sensitivity and tact You will need these skills as you support the home carer, the person who is dying and his relatives. Try not to intrude into their grief, and allow the home carer to do as much or as little of the caring as he or she wishes. Your role is to offer only the practical and psychological help that might be required of you. Allow friends and family as much privacy as you can. Respect their wishes at all times, particularly those who are religiously or spiritually motivated.

Sympathy and patience Empathise and be as sympathetic and patient as you can. Listen to the dying person's friends and relatives if they want to talk about their feelings; leave well alone if they do not.

Try to be patient when people repeat themselves, and show them that you are aware of their needs. If a person refuses to acknowledge what is happening, you should respect this.

Calmness and composure It is natural for grieving relatives to feel increasingly emotional and concerned as the dying person becomes weaker. You will need to remain calm at all times, particularly in the immediate period after the person has died, in order to provide comfort, reassurance and support.

SPIRITUAL AND CULTURAL NEEDS

You may be well aware of the dying person's spiritual views, but, if not, you may find it useful to acquaint yourself with his beliefs and customs.

Obtain information Ask the person, or his family and close friends, about his beliefs. Obtain additional information if needed.

Find out about religious customs Consult the spiritual adviser, if there is one, so that you are aware of any particular customs.

Show respect Once you are familiar with the person's spiritual needs, try to bear them in mind at all times.

Arrange special visits To gain the courage to face death, the person may ask you to arrange a visit from a member of his religious community, such as a priest.

REGISTERING A DEATH

It is the duty of a relative of the deceased who has knowledge of the particulars of the death to register the death within three months of the date of death.

THE REGISTRATION PROCESS

The registration of a death can take place at any Registration Office throughout the State. Copies of the Death Certificate may then be obtained from the registrar.

When attending a Civil Registration Office/ Private Registrar to register a death, the relative of the deceased, who must have identification, must ensure that they have the Death Registration Form completed by the Medical Practitioner who certified the death. There is no fee charged for the registration of a death. Fees are charged for copies of certificates.

LISTED BELOW ARE THE PARTICULARS WHICH WILL BE REGISTERED

- Full name, surname and sex;
- Former residence;
- Date of birth and age;
- Date and place where death occurred;
- Medical Certificate of Cause of Death signed by a registered Medical Practitioner who treated the deceased within 28 days before death. If the deceased was not seen by a doctor within 28 days or if he/she died as a result of an accident or in violent or mysterious circumstances the death must be referred to the coroner. A Post-Mortem examination may be required. The death can then be registered on foot of a certificate issued by the Coroner to the Registrar containing all the details;
- Personal Public Service Number (PPSN);
- Marital status;
- Occupation and occupation of spouse (if appropriate);
- Occupation of parent/guardian (if appropriate);
- Details of the Qualified Informant;
- Father of deceased name and surname;
- Mother of deceased name and maiden surname.

AFTER DEATH

The weeks that follow the death may prove to be difficult for you as you adjust from being a full-time carer. With less to occupy you, it is easy to dwell on your loss rather than look forward to the future. Now is the time for you to enjoy the company of people who care about you and those who miss your relative, and give and receive sympathy and support.

GRIEVING

While you may have anticipated the grief you would feel after losing a loved one, you may have grown accustomed to suppressing your feelings in the interests of caring for the person. Although it may be difficult, the ability to express your grief is an essential part of the recovery procedure. There are many ways you can help yourself through the grieving process.

Be patient Allow yourself the time to grieve.

Be open Try not to suppress your emotions. It is far healthier to shed tears and express your grief to others.

Be honest Do not feel guilty about being relieved or angry that your relative has died; these reactions often follow the loss of someone close, particularly if the person suffered, or you cared for her for a long time.

Be positive Try not to dwell solely on feelings of loss; try to use your grief positively by expressing the joy of having known your relative.

Be resourceful There are many organisations that provide advice and counselling; most hospices provide bereavement counselling.

GIVING AND RECEIVING SUPPORT

Grieving is a long process and it is important that support is maintained throughout this period. Sharing and exchanging sympathy can be a great comfort and will help all concerned to grieve.

Express yourself Try to express how you feel and how you intend to cope without the person.

Reminisce Be open: others may wish to talk to you about your relative and reminisce about the past.

Be sociable Make the effort to see people. If possible, try to maintain contact with those who have helped you; their continuing support may help you adjust to your new circumstances.

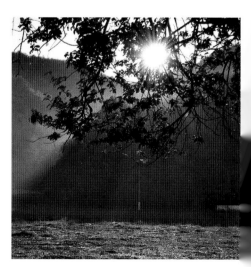

CHAPTER 14

USEFUL INFORMATION

The pages that follow aim to provide you with all the additional information that will be beneficial for you and your relative when dealing with issues such as the making of a will and the management of a persons financial affairs.

CONTENTS

MAKING A WILL

Most people have some property or money to leave after their death. No matter how small the amount, it is important to make a will in order to ensure that it goes where you want it. There are some restrictions on what you can do in a will. In general you may not completely disinherit a spouse and you must have fulfilled your obligations towards your children. Apart from that, you may dispose of your assets in whatever way you like.

Although it is advisable to get professional advice you may make a will yourself and it will be valid if you ensure that it is properly signed and that your signature is witnessed, by two people who are not beneficiaries under the will or married to a beneficiary under the will. If you have substantial property and/or money, you should definitely get professional advice. It is reasonable to enquire as to costs when engaging a solicitor.

THE REQUIREMENTS OF A VALID WILL

- the will must be in writing;
- you must be over 18 or have been or be married;
- you must be of sound mind;
- you must sign or mark the will or acknowledge the signature or mark in the presence of two witnesses. These two witnesses must be present with you simultaneously for their attestation to be valid; they must see you sign the will but they do not have to see the contents of the will;
- the signature or mark must be at the end of the will;
- the two witnesses must sign the will in your presence.

These are absolutely essential requirements and, if any one of them is not met, the will is not valid. If you subsequently want to change your will you may do so by adding a codicil (addition); this must meet exactly the same formal requirements as the will itself.

THE FORMAT OF THE WILL

It is not necessary that a will be in a set format. It is, however, recommended practice for the will to open by stating your name and address, followed by a clause revoking all earlier wills or codicils (additions) ('I hereby revoke all former wills and testamentary instruments made by me and declare this to be my last will and testament'), and a clause appointing executors (preferably more than one) and giving their addresses.

The will should then set out how you wish to dispose of your property and it is essential to include a residuary clause. A residuary clause is a clause setting out how property, which is not effectively dealt with in the will, should be disposed of. It is important as specific bequests may fail and the assets in question will revert to the 'residue'.

The will should then be dated, signed by the testator (person who makes a will), contain an attestation (evidence) clause which is usually expressed as follows 'Signed by the testator in the presence of us and by us in the presence of the testator' and be signed by the witnesses and their description and addresses set out. An attestation clause is not a formal requirement of a valid will but it is recommended because it constitutes evidence that the will has been validly executed.

WHERE THERE IS NO WILL

If a person dies without having made a will, or if the will is invalid for whatever reason, that person is said to have died 'intestate'. If there is a valid will but part of it is invalid then the part is dealt with as if there was intestacy. The rules for division of property on intestacy are as follows:

If the deceased is survived by:
- Spouse but no children (or grandchildren) - the spouse gets entire estate;
- Spouse and children - spouse gets two thirds, one third is divided equally between children (if a child has already died his/her children take the predeceased's child's share equally);
- Children, no spouse - divided equally between children (as above);
- Parents, no spouse or children - divided equally or entirely to one parent if only one survives;
- Brothers and sisters only - shared equally, the children of a deceased brother or sister take the share (if a child has already died his/her children take the predeceased's child's share equally);
- Nieces and nephews only - divided equally between those surviving;
- Other relatives - divided equally between nearest equal relationship;
- No relatives - the State.

On divorce, the spouse loses succession rights. However, when the court is assessing issues such as maintenance and property, it must take into account any benefit which either spouse loses as a result of the divorce.

INHERITANCE TAX

A properly drafted Will may help to reduce the amount charged in respect of Inheritance Tax. Capital Acquisitions Tax (CAT), which is both a tax on inheritance and on gifts, are both subject to self-assessment and it would be advisable to seek legal advice from your solicitor. The Revenue Commissioners will consider allowing the postponement of the tax due if there is hardship involved. In most cases, the payments may be spread over 5 years.

MANAGING SOMEONE'S FINANCES

You may have to oversee your relative's financial affairs if they are unable to manage them themselves. How this is done will depend entirely on their condition - that is, whether they are physically or mentally impaired - and their financial status. You should both seek independent legal advice before making any arrangements.

ENDURING POWER OF ATTORNEY

Power of Attorney authorises someone to act on behalf of another, usually in relation to their financial affairs, but also covering other matters. There are two types of Power of Attorney: a General Power of Attorney and an Enduring Power of Attorney. An Enduring Power of Attorney allows a person to choose in advance who will step into their shoes to deal with their financial affairs (and some personal decisions) in the event of them becoming mentally incapable (say, as a result of an accident or illness). An Enduring Power of Attorney can be executed out at any time, but it will only come into effect if the person becomes mentally incapable. At that stage, there is a registration procedure and the person who has been appointed as Power of Attorney can assume their role. The attorney does not have the power to make healthcare decisions.

JOINT PROPERTY AND ACCOUNTS

There are both advantages and disadvantages to putting property in joint names and your decision will depend on your particular circumstances. It is recommended that you seek legal advice from a solicitor before making any arrangements.

The legal position regarding ownership of assets including bank accounts is complex. It is important to take legal advice as to whether the balance of the account can be released to the survivor. For example, a bank account held by a husband and wife in joint names will usually (but not always) pass to the survivor, if one dies.

The position could be different for example, as between an uncle and niece.

CONTACT INFORMATION

IN CASE OF EMERGENCY DIAL 999 OR 112

RELATIVE/FRIEND
Name _____

Address _____

_____

_____

Phone _____

NEIGHBOUR
Name _____

Address _____

_____

_____

Phone _____

OTHER CARER
Name _____

Phone _____

GENERAL PRACTITIONER (GP)
Name _____

Address _____

_____

_____

Phone _____

PUBLIC HEALTH NURSE
Name _____

Address _____

_____

_____

Phone _____

OTHER CARE PROFESSIONALS
Name _____

Phone _____

WHERE IS IT?

GAS
Mains shut-off _____

ELECTRICITY
Fuse box _____

WATER
Mains tap _____

HEATING
Controls _____

Spare keys _____

Torch _____

Candles _____

GLOSSARY OF MEDICAL CONDITIONS

Abscess A collection of pus anywhere in the body. A boil is a common type of abscess.

AIDS (Acquired Immune Deficiency Syndrome). A condition in which the immune system stops functioning properly. It is caused by infection with HIV (human immunodeficiency virus), which is transmitted sexually and through the blood.

Alzheimer's Disease A name given to forms of dementia (see Dementia) not resulting from disease of the brain's blood vessels. It results in loss of memory, confusion and unpredictable behaviour.

Anaemia A deficiency of haemoglobin, the red pigment in blood cells that carries oxygen around the body. The most usual cause is lack of iron. Symptoms include pallor and fatigue.

Angina Chest pain caused by narrowing of the blood vessels that supply the heart. When the demand for oxygen is increased, for example, during exercise or stress, the affected heart does not receive enough oxygen, leading to pain.

Arthritis Inflammation of the joints. The joints, especially the protective capsule, become diseased or worn out causing varying degrees of pain and disability. Two common types of arthritis are osteoarthritis and rheumatoid arthritis.

Asthma Attacks of wheezing and breathlessness, which can become severe. It is caused by narrowing of the airways and is often triggered by allergy or an infection, e.g. to pollen or to house dust.

Bronchitis Inflammation of the bronchi, the larger airways of the lungs. Common symptoms are breathlessness, coughing, and production of phlegm. Acute bronchitis is usually shortlived and commonly follows a viral illness such as a cold, or inhalation of an irritant substance. Repeated attacks may result in chronic bronchitis, a permanent condition seen especially in smokers and those exposed repeatedly to air pollution.

Cancer A malignant tumour (growth), which if untreated, can be fatal. Tumours can develop in any organ of the body, interfering with their function and destroying healthy tissue. Cells from the tumour can travel to other parts of the body to form secondary growths.

Cataract A disorder of the lens of the eye. The lens becomes opaque (milky in appearance), reducing the amount of light entering the eye. It may result in blindness.

Cerebral Palsy Poor coordination and abnormal muscular control of various parts of the body due to brain damage, which most commonly takes place at birth.

Chickenpox An illness caused by a virus varicella zoster. Often described as a childhood illness, adults can also contract it. Symptoms include a high temperature, headache, and a red rash from which small blisters develop. The blisters are extremely irritating, but if they or their scabs are picked, scarring can result.

Conjunctivitis Inflammation of the conjunctiva, the membrane that covers the front of the eye. It causes redness, itching and discharge from the eye.

Coronary Thrombosis A blood clot in the arteries supplying the heart. It can occur suddenly, usually in arteries narrowed by disease. If the clot fails to dissolve quickly, part of the heart muscle dies, causing a heart attack (myocardial infarction). It is accompanied by severe central chest pain perhaps travelling to the neck and left arm, with profound shock and a feeling of doom.

Cystic Fibrosis An inherited disorder that is usually present at birth. It affects various glands and is characterised by secretion of sticky mucus, repeated chest infections and failure to grow properly due to poor digestion of food.

Cystitis An acute inflammation of the bladder. Often caused by an infection, it causes lower abdominal pain together with painful and frequent passing of urine.

Dementia Gradual loss of intellect due to progressive deterioration of the brain cells. It is sometimes the result of deterioration of the brain's blood vessels and is usually, but not always, confined to the elderly. Dementia causes anxiety, memory loss and confusion.

Depression (depressive illness) An excessive down-swing of mood sometimes accompanied by lack of appetite, sleep disturbance and fatigue. Its seriousness is often underestimated and medical advice should be sought.

Dermatitis Inflammation of the skin, a variety of which is known as eczema. It results in red, shiny, dry, cracked areas of skin. Scratching causes infection and weeping skin.

Diabetes A condition resulting from the pancreas secreting insufficient insulin. Symptoms include excessive thirst, frequent urination, weight loss, and in severe cases, it can lead to coma.

Eczema See Dermatitis.

Emphysema A disease of the lungs in which the small air sacs (alveoli) are destroyed. It causes breathlessness and can lead to heart failure. Often caused by smoking, emphysema also commonly accompanies chronic bronchitis and severe long-term asthma.

Epilepsy A condition in which periods of abnormal electrical activity in the brain can lead to seizures, loss of consciousness and possibly convulsions.

Gastroenteritis Inflammation of the stomach and bowel leading to diarrhoea and vomiting. It is normally due to a virus or eating contaminated food. Most cases will settle in 24 to 48 hours, but the condition can be more serious if the sufferer is very young or elderly, or if the symptoms are severe or prolonged.

Glandular Fever A viral infection, which characteristically results in swelling of the glands in the neck (lymph nodes). Other symptoms include high temperature and a sore throat.

Glaucoma A condition in which pressure builds up in the eyeball. It can lead to permanent damage and blindness.

Haemophilia A hereditary disease that affects males only, in which the blood fails to clot due to a lack of an ingredient known as Factor Eight.

Heart Attack See Coronary thrombosis.

Hepatitis Inflammation of the liver with a range of causes such as alcohol, medication and viruses. Viral hepatitis types A and E are transmitted mostly through drinking water contaminated by infected faeces. Hepatitis types B, C and D are transmitted through blood and sexual contact.

Herpes Simplex A virus responsible for cold sores and genital herpes. It causes small blisters that erupt in the skin.

Herpes Zoster See Shingles.

Influenza (flu) An acute viral infection. Symptoms include high fever, sweating and muscle aches. In a healthy adult, the illness runs its course in seven to ten days and a full recovery usually results. Pneumonia is a dangerous complication, occurring more frequently in young children and the elderly.

Laryngitis Inflammation of the larynx (voice box). It results in a sore throat, cough and a hoarse or lost voice. Laryngitis is commonly associated with infections of the upper and lower respiratory tract but can also occur after misuse of the voice.

Leukaemia A cancer (see Cancer) that affects the white cells in the blood.

Measles An infectious disease caused by a virus. It has an incubation period of 7 to 14 days. It initially presents with a raised temperature and watery eyes and nose. A light pink rash develops which becomes more extensive over 3 to 4 days. There is no cure and treatment is aimed at relieving symptoms. There are a number of possible serious complications including pneumonia and brain damage. There is an effective vaccine available.

Meningitis A bacterial or viral infection that causes inflammation of the protective membranes (meninges) that surround the brain. Symptoms include severe headaches, avoidance of light, neck stiffness, nausea, vomiting and confusion and, in some cases, a reddish-purple rash. Bacterial meningitis can be severe and life threatening.

Motor Neurone Disease A progressive disease affecting the nerves that control muscular activity. It usually appears in older people and results in increasing disability.

MRSA (Methicillin or multi resistant Staphaureus) A bacteria that has become resistant to many of the more common antibiotics making its treatment and eradication difficult. It is a particular problem in hospitals for patients following surgery or who are immunocompromised. The key to preventing its spread is good hygiene. It may be present in a healthy individual (particularly in the nose) in the community without causing difficulty.

Multiple Sclerosis A disease affecting the sheaths that protect particular nerves in the brain and spinal cord. It usually begins in early adulthood and progresses gradually with remissions. It causes weakness, poor coordination, loss of sensation and eye and bladder disturbances. Mood changes are common.

Mumps An infectious disease caused by a virus characterised by a swelling of the salivary glands in the face principally in front of the ears. The incubation period is 16 to 21 days. There is no cure and treatment is aimed at relieving symptoms. There are a number of possible serious complications including meningitis. There is an effective vaccine available.

Muscular Dystrophy A group of hereditary disorders affecting the muscles (but not the nerves). They commonly affect children, causing progressive weakness and consequent deformities.

Osteoporosis A condition in which bone loses its density. When severe, it can lead to fractures occuring easily or even spontaneously (without any trauma). Hormones have a strong influence on bone density and osteoporosis more commonly occurs in women after the menopause when the level of the oestrogen hormone is reduced.

Parkinson's Disease A disease of the central nervous system. Due to lack of certain chemical substances in the brain, there is a progressive onset of muscular tremors and rigidity. Characteristic signs include trembling hands, slow speech and a stiff, shuffling walk. It usually occurs in the elderly.

Pneumonia An acute infection of the lungs. It is characterised by high fever, shivering and the production of infected green or yellow phlegm, which may be bloodstained. Bacteria usually cause the infection.

Polio A viral illness, which in a minority of cases damages the motor nerves in the spinal cord causing a paralysis of a limb or even of the muscles involved in breathing. Vaccination has now virtually eradicated the disease in many countries.

Rheumatism A commonly used term for joint and muscular aches and pains.

Rubella Also known as German Measles, is caused by a virus. It has an incubation period of 14 to 21 days and usually presents with a light pink rash that lasts for three days. It can cause foetal abnormalities if a woman gets the infection during the first three months of pregnancy. There is an effective vaccine available.

Scabies A skin infestation caused by a mite. It is spread by direct skin-to-skin contact. The mite burrows into the skin and causes an allergic reaction with intense irritation. Common sites affected are the finger-webs, wrists, elbows, armpits, the groin area and buttocks.

Shingles Following an episode of chickenpox the virus remains dormant in the person's body in the nerves near the spinal cord. At some point the virus may become reactivated causing a blistering painful rash on the skin. The rash will only appear in a strip corresponding to the area supplied by the nerve in which it became reactivated. The risk of another person getting chickenpox from a person with shingles is extremely low.

Sinusitis Inflammation of the sinuses (air-filled cavities around the nose). It is caused by an allergy or by an infection and it may also follow a cold. Symptoms include pain behind the cheeks and the upper jaw. A build-up of fluid occurs which, if infected by bacteria, causes fever and the production of yellow-green mucus.

Spina Bifida A defect present at birth in which one or more vertebrae has not developed completely and the spinal cord is exposed. It results in varying degrees of disability. Infection within the spinal canal is the most serious complication.

Stoma An opening in the body created surgically. If the voice box is removed, a stoma is created at the front of the neck through which the patient can breathe. Stomas are also made in the abdomen to collect faeces in patients with intestinal diseases.

Stroke Damage to the brain caused by a blood clot or haemorrhage. It can result in loss of consciousness or even coma, loss of speech and other bodily functions, and varying degrees of paralysis of different parts of the body.

Thrombosis A blood clot inside a blood vessel. If the thrombosis occurs in the brain, heart or lung, the person's life may be at risk. A clot forming in the leg may not be life threatening in itself, but part of it may break off and travel to the lungs.

Tuberculosis (TB) An infectious, airborne disease that usually affects the lungs, causing coughing, chest pain and fever.

Whooping Cough (Pertusis) A highly infectious disease caused by Bordetella Pertusis. It is characterised by severe bouts of coughing followed by an inspiratory whooping noise and often vomiting. 90% of cases are in children under 5 years. The incubation period is 7 to 14 days. Treatment with antibiotics may only limit the severity of the disease. Complications may include pneumonia, convulsions and chronic lung damage. There is an effective vaccine available.

TUBE FEEDING

Tube Feeding also known as enteral feeding, refers to any method of nutrient ingestion via the gastrointestinal tract and may be considered in patients who have a functional gastrointestinal tract but cannot obtain nutrition by swallowing. It may be temporary in treatment of acute conditions, or lifelong in the case of chronic disabilities. A variety of tubes are used in medical practise, usually made of polyurethane or silicone. The diameter of a feeding tube is measured in French units; and is classified by site of insertion and intended use.

TYPES OF ENTERAL FEEDING TUBES

Nasogastric - The most commonly used tube feed. The nasogastric feeding tube, NG-tube, is passed through the nostrils down the oesophagus and into the stomach and may be weighted to hold position. This type of feeding is generally used for short term feeding, ten to fourteen days maximum.

Gastric - A gastric feeding tube (G-tube) is inserted through a small incision in the abdomen into the stomach and is used for long term enteral nutrition. The percutaneous endoscopic gastrostomy (PEG) tube is one kind and is placed endoscopically. A needle is inserted through the abdomen, visualised within the stomach by the endoscope. The insertion of the tube takes about twenty minutes and kept within the stomach either by a balloon on its tip (which can be deflated) or by a retention dome.

The G-T and the PEG-tube are suitable for long - term use; and are used where there is difficulty with swallowing (dysphagia) stroke victims and concerns of aspiration pneumonia.

Jejunostomy - For patients with gastric disease this may be the more suitable feeding route. A jejunostomy feeding tube (J-tube) is a tube surgically inserted through the abdomen and into the jejunum (the second part of the intestine).

ENTERAL FEEDS

The administration of enteral feeds may be via gravity drip or pump assisted. They are commercially prepared, sterile available as liquid or powder and have the advantage of being of known composition. So they can be tailored to suit the patient's requirements.

Complications may occur but the overall rate is low. They may include irritation around the site of insertion. The use of barrier creams, dressings and frequent cleaning is generally recommended to prevent this. A very rare but serious complication would be leakage from the punctured hole in the stomach into the abdomen causing severe infection and death.

HOME DIALYSIS

Kidney Function is essential to sustain life. Once a patient's kidneys show signs of failure the doctor or nurse will discuss the options available. These will include Dialysis. Kidney (Renal) dialysis is used when a patient has either suddenly lost kidney function or has chronic kidney disease that gradually causes the kidneys to fail; it is a process in which the blood is filtered to remove waste products and the excess fluid that builds up because the kidneys are not working properly.

There are two types of treatment: **Haemodialysis** and **Peritoneal** dialysis. They remove waste and excess water from the blood in different ways.

Haemodialysis removes waste and water by circulating blood outside the body through an external filter containing a membrane and a dialysate (special dialysis fluid). This is a more rigorous treatment and requires close attention from the medical team, usually its hospital based. However if this is the chosen option it can be operated at home. Prior to commencing Home Haemodialysis (HHD), the service adviser will arrange:

- The required tests, patient admission to hospital to create an access point from which the blood can be safely removed and returned to the body. The two main types of access are; arteriovenous fistula, (AV fistula) and central venous catheter (CV catheter.)
- Training in care of; AV fistula/CV catheter and self needling.
- House conversion; creating electricity supply, water and drainage in the designated room.
- Organise and setup the required equipment which includes: Home Haemodialysis Machine. Dialysis chair

and table .Weighing scales. Waste disposal equipment including a sharps bin, healthcare risk waste bags and wheelie bin.

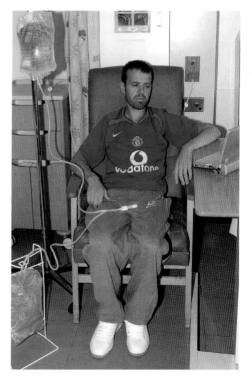

Supervision and support is provided by the home therapy nurse. This is an ideal therapy for patients waiting a prolonged time for, or who are unsuitable for kidney transplant the advantages include:

- Not needing to travel to hospital three times a week for dialysis
- Having the dialysis when it suits, as discussed with the home dialysis team
- Choosing to have longer dialysis sessions and more frequent than three times weekly. An added benefit to health allowing more flexibility in the renal diet.
- Patient has more control of their condition

Some disadvantages to HHD therapy include:
- Setting up and dismantling the dialysis machine for each treatment
- Designating a space in the patients home for the storage of the dialysis equipment

Peritoneal Dialysis (PD) takes place inside the body. The peritoneum is a layer of tissue containing blood vessels that lines and surrounds the abdominal cavity and internal abdominal organs, stomach, spleen liver and intestines. A sterile solution containing glucose at body temperature is run through a tube (Tenckoff catheter) into the peritoneal cavity. The peritoneal membrane (peritoneum) acts as a partial permeable membrane to filter the waste products and excess fluid from the blood into the fluid in the peritoneum. The Tenckhoff catheter is inserted into the peritoneal cavity by way of a minor operation then it is allowed to rest for a period of weeks before it can be used.

Continuous Ambulant Peritoneal Dialysis (CAPD) Dialysis fluid at room temperature, is instilled into the peritoneal cavity four times a day via the Tenckoff catheter. Different strengths of dialysis are available. The doctor and the PD nurse will explain and advise the best suited to the patient. This fluid is left in the patient's abdomen cavity - for an agreed period, waste products and the extra fluid moves from the patients blood into the peritoneal space and are drained out through the catheter and discarded fresh solution instilled, which takes approximately 30 minutes. This cycle or 'exchange' is normally repeated 4-5 times during the day and operated by gravity.

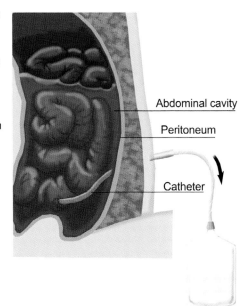

Abdominal cavity

Peritoneum

Catheter

Automated Peritoneal Dialysis (APD)

APD is an overnight treatment ranging from 10-12 hours, and involves the use of a machine to perform the dialysis while the patient sleeps. A small volume of fluid remains in the abdomen all day and at night when connected to the machine the fluid is removed and replaced at intervals

Complications of Peritoneal Dialysis
- Peritonitis: Inflammation of the peritoneum
- Exit site infection.
- Fluid leak.
- Inadequate dialysis.
- Catheter blockage

Peritonitis is the most serious and most common complication of peritoneal dialysis. CCPD provides a little more protection against peritonitis than CAPD because it requires the closed, sterile dialysis system to be interrupted less frequently. To reduce the risk of peritonitis, patients using either form of peritoneal dialysis should practice meticulous hand hygiene when connecting and disconnecting their catheter to the dialysate. Observation of the Tenchkoff exit site for any indications of infection is required daily and any concerns reported to the PD staff immediately.

As PD is carried out at home by the patient, it does free the patient from the routine of attending dialysis clinic three times a week. With peritoneal dialysis, diet is usually less restrictive than with haemodialysis because waste removal is continuous rather than intermittent. Because each renal replacement therapy option has the potential to affect all aspects of a patient's life, individuals need to make the choice that's compatible with their lifestyle. It's also important that patients understand that in choosing a method, they're not necessarily committing to that method for life. As patients' health status or social situation changes, it may be appropriate for them to reconsider their options and make a different renal replacement therapy choice

INDEX

NOTES